CW00956760

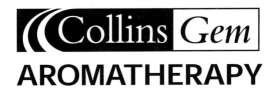

AROMATHERAPY

Lucinda Deacon-Davis

HarperCollins*Publishers*

Lucinda Deacon-Davis (I.T.E.C, SWS Dip. (Aroma), A.O.C. Reg, M.A.H.P. (Int), I.I.H.H.T, C&G Teach. Cert.) is a qualified holistic therapist specialising in aromatherapy, massage and reflexology.

HarperCollins Publishers
Westerhill Road, Bishopbriggs, Glasgow G64 2QT

Devised and created by The Printer's Devil, Glasgow

First published 2001

Reprint 10 9 8 7 6 5 4 3 2 1 0

ISBN 0 00 710146 5

Photocredits
Graham Lees pp. 7, 14, 19, 20, 27, 42, 42, 43, 45, 47, 50, 53, 57, 60, 68, 69, 70, 71, 77, 79, 81, 83, 84, 85, 89, 91, 94, 95, 97, 98, 104, 115, 117, 120, 123, 127, 128, 130, 143, 146, 162
PS5 pp. 30, 39, 44, 48, 56, 79, 83, 91, 97, 106, 113, 115, 131, 132, 142, 163-179
Artville © pp. 10, 21, 44, 47, 52, 56, 61, 64, 67, 68, 71, 74, 78, 83, 87, 90, 93, 96, 102, 106, 109, 113, 117, 119, 122
Photodisc © pp. 12, 25, 29, 31, 32, 44, 48, 53, 57, 61, 62, 64, 65, 68, 71, 75, 79, 83, 84, 87, 88, 90, 93, 97, 98, 103, 106, 107, 109, 110, 114, 115, 118, 119, 144, 150, 181, 182, 184, 185
Harry Smith Horticultural Photographic Collection © pp. 51, 55, 63, 73, 100, 134
A–Z Botanical Collection Ltd © pp. 59, 92, 108, 116, 134

The Printer's Devil would like to thank Quinessence Aromatherapy for the image of the Denza Blue Aromastone, p. 23, and the Australian Government for the image of the tea tree on p. 112

Printed in Italy by Amadeus S.p.A.

CONTENTS

INTRODUCTION

This book explains what aromatherapy is all about
and how you can safely use this therapy on yourself,
family and friends to bring about many health
benefits.

A range of the most useful essential oils is included
along with their benefits and how you can enjoy the
wide range of aromas from these oils.

Quick reference sections make it easy to select
essential oils for benefits while at work, at home and
on holiday. Sections on veterinary usage of the oils
and use of aromatherapy in pregnancy and with
children are also included.

WHAT IS AROMATHERAPY?

The definition of aromatherapy is 'the safe use of essential oils for therapeutic benefits, enhancing the well-being, restoring balance and revitalising the mind, body and spirit'. In other words, essential oils – which come from plants – are used safely in a way to promote general good health and well-being.

THE HISTORY OF AROMATHERAPY

Since ancient times, plants have been used to heal, fight infection, aid digestion and promote well-being. From prehistoric times through Ancient Egyptians and the Arab world, knowledge of the healing properties of plants came to the West via the Crusaders.

Herbalism and aromatherapy were neglected by advances in modern science and medicine until their rediscovery by European scientists in the 1920s and '30s, but since the 1970s aromatherapy in Britain has boomed, taking its place in mainstream alternative and conventional therapies.

WHAT ARE ESSENTIAL OILS?

Essential oils are a form of plant essence, and are extracted mainly by steam distillation from plants. They can come from any part of the plant: from the petals, as with rose, jasmine, or neroli; the root, with ginger; leaves with tea tree; tree resin for frankincense; and even the wood itself, to produce sandalwood.

Although they are called oils, essential oils are in fact similar in substance to water or alcohol, with some, like sandalwood, being slightly thicker in consistency.

These oils are highly concentrated and they contain all the important therapeutic properties of the plant material including the aroma of the plants in a very highly concentrated state. With some oils, many tons of plant material are needed to produce only a small amount of essential oil, such as rose and neroli oil. This can make the oils quite expensive, although only a few drops are needed in aromatherapy.

All the oils have important therapeutic properties: some are sedative, others uplifting, some diuretic, others anti-inflammatory, most are antiseptic, some are very effective at fighting viral or fungal infections and yet others can have an effect on the hormonal system.

The oils are always diluted and can be used in a maximum combination of three at a time. In many cases they are more effective when used in a blend as opposed to being used on their own. Essential oils can heal on both an emotional and physical level.

How To Use Essential Oils

There are three methods of using the oils:

- absorption through the skin as in massage or bathing
- absorption through the nose by inhalation
- ingestion, through the stomach (*not* recommended).

It is advisable not to take any essential oils internally because the highly concentrated nature of the essential oils could cause severe damage to the stomach lining.

HOW DOES AROMATHERAPY WORK?

Aromatherapy works by the absorption of the essential oils through the skin or through the nose, into the blood stream and then to various areas of the body. (See p. 8 on the dangers of ingesting.)

Sense of Smell

Inhalation of essential oil is the quickest method of penetration and the mechanism of smell in the body is one of the oldest senses that we have. We do not use our sense of smell as much as our forebears did, who would have relied on it when hunting for food and for warnings of approaching danger.

But our sense of smell is still very important as it gives taste to our food and it has a strong effect on our emotions. Think of the effect of smelling freshly cut grass or freshly mowed hay, reminding you of summer. Or how the smell of an aftershave or perfume will bring back memories of a loved one. These reactions are almost instantaneous, so it is easy to see how fast the aroma of an essential oil can affect how we feel.

Our sense of smell varies from one person to another and at different times. The strongest sense of smell is in a woman at ovulation and in pregnancy.

THROUGH THE NOSE

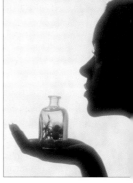

The sense of smell is thought to be linked to the limbic system, an old part of the brain. When you add essential oils to a bath or a burner, the oils' molecules are released into the air around you. You then inhale these through the nose.

At the top of the nose are little hairs called cilia; these have tiny indentations. As the essential oil molecules pass over the hairs they fit into the indentations like a key in a lock; this then sets off a signal to the brain via the olfactory bulb. The signal is sent to the limbic system and other important parts of the brain, causing a reaction in the nervous system. The reaction caused is dependent on the type of aroma smelt, and this in turn might cause a relaxing or stimulating response on a part of the body.

This reaction or nervous signal, can also have physical effect on the body; for instance, in the form of pain relief, by stimulating the endocrine system or boosting the immune system.

Inhalation of essential oils is the quickest method of application, having an effect on the brain within minutes, which in turn has an immediate effect on the

DIFFERENT METHODS OF INHALATION

- electric diffuser
- aromatherapy burner
- light bulb rings
- aromastones
- in a bath
- in a steam room
- in a sauna
- air sprays
- drops on a tissue
- added to a pot pourri
- from a bowl (steam inhalation)
- inhale from a drop of oil in the hands

emotions. When inhaling, the oils are in direct contact with the mucus membrane on the inside of the nose and the lungs, so this is the most useful method for complaints such as catarrh, sinusitis, etc.

THROUGH THE SKIN

The skin is a semi-permeable membrane, which will allow for the passage of certain substances in and out of the body; for instance, salts are removed from the body by sweat through the pores. Medication, such as HRT patches and nicotine patches are used as a slow way of administering drugs into the body via the skin.

Essential oils, which are very small particles or molecules, get into the body in the same way. Once through the skin, the molecules are absorbed into the blood stream and lymph system, then they are carried to various parts of the body.

This process can take from 20 minutes to several hours depending on the skin type of the individual. If skin is dry and healthy, then the oils will be absorbed quickly; but if the person is a heavy smoker or has a skin complaint the process can be a lot slower, as the body is pushing out toxins which will hinder the passage of the essential oils. The same is true of anyone sweating heavily and expelling salts and fluids.

ABSORPTION

The main method of absorption used in aromatherapy is by massage, and this is the method commonly used by aromatherapists.

Due to their concentrated nature, the essential oils are firstly diluted in a vegetable carrier oil, like sweet almond or grapeseed. It is important that a vegetable oil is used, as a mineral oil like baby oil will sit on the surface of the skin and form a barrier to the penetration of essential oils.

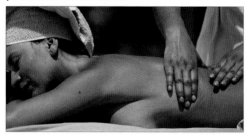

DIFFERENT METHODS OF ABSORPTION

- in a bath
- sitz bath
- Jacuzzis
- gargle
- diluted in a carrier oil for massage
- in a compress (hot or cold)

EFFECTS ON THE BODY

Pharmacologically Firstly, they can affect the body chemically by reacting with its hormones and enzymes.

Certain essential oils like fennel contain a natural form of oestrogen and they appear to mimic the effect of oestrogen in the body, making this oil useful for menopausal and menstrual irregularities. Other oils like tea tree appear to increase the production of the white blood corpuscles so important for our immune system, so tea tree is a useful oil to help fight infection.

Physiologically Secondly, they can cause an overall stimulating or sedating reaction in the body.

Basil is a useful stimulant and ideal for study, while lavender has an overall sedating effect on the body.

Psychologically Thirdly, and one of the most important ways, is by influencing the emotions.

Most essential oils have this ability: some, like bergamot are uplifting, and so ideal for depression; sandalwood is an aphrodisiac so will sexually stimulate the body; and ginger is very warming and comforting, and is good to use when feeling lonely.

ESSENTIAL OILS & THEIR EXTRACTION

PRECIOUS ESSENCES

Essential oils are a form of essence extracted from various parts of a plant – flower petals from a rose, leaves in eucalyptus, the rind of citrus fruit and sometimes the roots or rhizomes, as with ginger.

These very aromatic plant essences, or essential oils, are found in oil glands in plant tissue and seem to have important functions. It is thought the oils help to attract beneficial insects while deterring those that would harm it, so the plant has its own natural insecticide. The oils also seem to protect the plant from bacteria and fungal infection. These oils form the life force of the plant and it is possible that the scent is used as a form of communication between plants.

The properties of these plant essences are not lost during the extraction process: in many ways they seem to be enhanced, forming concentrated essential oils.

As explained in What Is Aromatherapy? (p. 6), most oils are more like water or alcohol in consistency and are generally colourless to pale yellow. Essential oils are nearly always diluted, mainly in a vegetable carrier

APPLYING ESSENTIAL OILS

Essential oils can be applied in many ways to get the full benefit of their exquisite aroma and therapeutic powers. The use of oils in massage or in a vaporiser or burner are particularly popular, but oils can be incorporated into everyday life in many more ways.

Due to their concentrated nature, some type of carrier is needed to apply the oils. This can be as simple as air, when using burners, vaporisers or steam inhalation; water when using the oils in a bath; or vegetable oil, in the case of massage.

AIR AS A CARRIER

Using air as a carrier, there are many ways that essential oils can be used in order to inhale their aroma to get the quickest effect and the maximum benefit of their powers.

From your hands Put a drop of essential oil on your palms, rub your hands together, cup them over your nose and inhale. This simple method can be carried out anywhere, at any time.

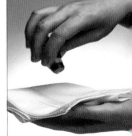

From a handkerchief Place a couple of drops of

essential oil on a tissue or handkerchief, sniff it by taking three deep breaths, then tuck the tissue in your blouse or shirt and the warmth of your body will continue to give off the oil's aroma. Be careful not to use oils which could stain clothes or irritate the skin.

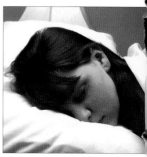

Drops on a pillow To help you sleep, put a couple of drops of lavender or camomile on either side of your pillow; you will still smell the oil when turning over in the night.

Steam inhalation This method comes into its own in winter when colds and flu abound. To a basin of hot water, add 2–3 drops of essential oil, ideally peppermint or eucalyptus, put a towel over your head and lean over the bowl inhaling deeply. Repeat until the water goes cold or the oils evaporate. Do this two or three times a day to help relieve the symptoms of colds, flu, headaches, blocked sinuses and hayfever. (This is *not* recommended for asthma sufferers.)

FRAGRANCING ROOMS

Pot pourri Put dried or fresh flower petals in a bowl and sprinkle on your favourite essential oils to give a lovely fresh fragrance to a room.

Air spray freshener Half-fill a plastic plant-spray bottle with water (250 ml) and add 6–10 drops of a refreshing essential oil. Shake the bottle and spray for a quick, and environmentally friendly air freshener. (Do not spray directly on polished furniture.)

Vaporiser or burner A traditional way of fragrancing a room with essential oil. Vaporisers come in different materials, from terracotta to porcelain or even metal, all with two separate containers: the top one for water and essential oils, and the bottom one housing a night-light candle. Try to get one with a large top reservoir that does not need constant topping up, and ideally one with separate containers for easy cleaning.

Light the candle in the bottom container, into the top container add water and 6–8 drops of essential oil, depending on the size of the room. As the water warms, the essential oils will start to evaporate and their aroma will be dissipated.

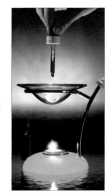

This is an inexpensive way to fragrance a room, but be careful: you are using a naked flame and the water in the vaporiser will get quite hot. If there are children, pets or elderly people in the vicinity you may want to consider using an electric diffuser instead.

Electric diffusers These are much safer than candle-heated vaporisers but they can be expensive. There are many different types and they can be purchased from large chemists, health-food shops or aromatherapy suppliers.

Some have a felt pad on which you add a few drops of essential oil, and an electrically heated element or a fan underneath causes the oils to evaporate into the air. Others rely on the vibration of the essential oils to disperse them, assisted by cool air. This type uses no heat.

These diffusers can be used overnight or in an office environment.

Aromastones These vaporisers are safer than the candle-heated variety., and can be left unattended and switched on overnight.

The heavy ceramic stone-shaped vaporiser is heated

FRAGRANCING ROOMS

- To freshen or deodorise a room, use peppermint, lemon, grapefruit and other refreshing oils

- To disinfect a room, use eucalyptus, lavender, tea tree and rosemary

- To give an uplifting atmosphere, use geranium and citrus oils

- To repel insects, use lavender, lemon, eucalyptus, peppermint or geranium

electrically and a slight indentation in the stone allows you to add a little water and a few drops of essential oil. (You can also use the oils on their own if you prefer.) When the 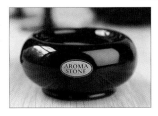 stone is switched on, it heats up to vaporise the oils. Aromastones are easy to clean. They are available from aromatherapy suppliers, but if you are buying one, try to get the type that has a light to indicate when it is switched on.

Light-bulb rings These grooved rings are made of ceramic or metal and oils are added to the groove and then placed on top of a light bulb. When the light bulb is switched on, the heat emitted from the bulb will diffuse the oils into the atmosphere.

Put 2–3 drops of your chosen oil into the groove of the ring (*do not* add water), place the ring on a light bulb and switch on the light. Make sure that the light bulb is cold before using a light-bulb ring and never add essential oils directly to a light bulb.

Light-bulb rings are a very cheap way to vaporise essential oils and are available from health-food shops and aromatherapy suppliers. They are ideal for use at night to fragrance a room before going to bed, and safe enough to use in a child's or elderly person's room.

Radiating aroma Radiator diffusers are specially designed to fit on radiators. Water and a few drops of essential oil are added to a small bowl in the diffuser which is then hooked onto a radiator. The radiator's heat causes the oils to vaporise. This is a cheap and fairly safe way to fragrance a room with oils, but it needs to kept out of the reach of children and pets.

Alternatively, using a ball of cotton wool, sprinkle on a few drops of essential oils and place behind a radiator. Do not let the oils come in direct contact with the radiator as the metal and paint may be damaged by the essential oils over a period of time.

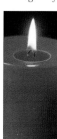

Aromatherapy candles An attractive way to fragrance a room. Genuine aromatherapy candles are available from specialist candle shops or aromatherapy suppliers, or you could make your own (see *Using Essential Oils at Home*, p. 122). Some of those more widely available are often merely fragranced with synthetic perfume.

As always with candles, care must be taken in use.

WATER AS A CARRIER

Although essential oils do not readily dissolve in water, the use of water as a medium in aromatherapy is very beneficial.

BATHING
BENEFITS

One of the
most relaxing
ways to use
essential oils
is in the bath.
This has a
double bene-
fit as the oils
are inhaled as
well as being
absorbed via
the skin. It is
a useful

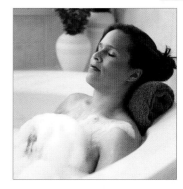

method of using essential oils to benefit aching
muscles, skin problems and to help you sleep.

Aromatic baths Essential oils can be added straight
to the bath water, but if you have sensitive skin or this
is the first time you have used a particular essential oil
in the bath, you should dilute the essential oil first.

To do this, add 7–10 drops of essential oil to a small
amount of vegetable oil, or pretend you are Cleopatra
for a moment and dilute the essential oils in full-fat
milk! (Skimmed milk won't work.) Full-fat milk
powder can also be used: add the essential oils to a
little milk powder, add some water to form a paste.

Once the essential oils are dissolved in the milk or

vegetable oil they can be added to the bath. It is important to run the bath first, then add the diluted oils and swish them around in the water. If you add the oils to a running bath they will evaporate before you have chance to get their full benefit.

If you are using the oil neat, add 7–10 drops once the bath has been run and swish them around in the water before getting in. Soak in the bath for 10 minutes before using any soap or bubble bath, as these synthetic products will cancel out the therapeutic effects of the essential oils.

Sitz bath A sitz bath with essential oils is a very useful way of dealing with complaints like haemorrhoids, stitches after childbirth, thrush and cystitis. Put 3–4 drops of a suitable oil, for example tea tree for thrush, into a bowl of warm water and sit in it for 10 minutes.

Foot bath For aching feet or foot disorders like athlete's foot and blisters, put 4–6 drops of essential oil in a bowl and soak the feet for 10 minutes. Tea tree is beneficial for blisters and athlete's foot, while peppermint is excellent for tired feet.

Showers Don't worry if you only have a shower at home – you can still benefit from the effects of essential oils. Put 4–6 drops of essential oil on a sponge or face cloth while in the shower and rub briskly over the body. The aroma of the oils will be released by the heat of the water, enabling you to inhale them. This method can be used as a refreshing treatment, particularly if using citrus oils.

Epsom salts bath An Epsom salts bath is an excellent way of detoxing the body particularly in cases of arthritis, aching muscles and colds or flu.

You can buy industrial Epsom salts (magnesium sulphate) from the chemist. Dissolve 450 grams in a few pints of boiling water then add to the bath and soak for 15 minutes. Essential oils can be added to the bath.

Do not have an Epsom salts bath if you have high blood pressure or a heart condition. Move any arthritic joints as much as possible after the bath to prevent toxins collecting in the joints.

COMPRESSES

Hot or cold compresses are an invaluable way to treat conditions such as period pain, stomach aches, muscle strains, headaches, arthritic joints, varicose veins and burns. If the problem involves heat or inflammation a cold compress is best, but if there is a dull ache, use a hot compress.

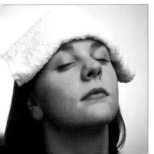

Hot compress To prepare, take a small towel or flannel and soak in a bowl of 500 ml of hot water which contains 5–6 drops of essential oil. Wring out the cloth and apply to the affected area and replace when the compress becomes cold.

Use a hot compress with clary sage for period pains and with marjoram for stomach aches, when the compress should be applied to the tummy. Place a hot compress with marjoram on the back of the neck in cases of migraine.

Cold compress A cold compress is particularly beneficial for headaches – place on the forehead; sprains and strains – place on the injured area; and burns and sunburn – use a cold compress with lavender.

To prepare a cold compress, put cold water (add ice if a strain or sprain) in a bowl, add 5–6 drops of essential oil and soak a towel or flannel in the bowl. Apply to affected part and leave for between 20 minutes and an hour (keep re-soaking the compress in the water).

Hot & cold When arthritis flares up and there are hot, swollen or inflamed joints, it is not advisable to massage, but instead use alternating hot and cold compresses to bring relief. Apply each compress for 2–3 minutes and repeat the cycle of hot and cold two or three times, ending with a cold compress.

Gargle & mouth wash For instant relief from a sore throat, mouth ulcer, loss of voice, bad breath or laryngitis, try gargling with tea tree. Its antiseptic properties make it very effective at tackling any mouth or throat infection.

To gargle, add 2 drops (no more) to half a glass of warm water or cider vinegar and gargle, making sure you spit out afterwards. If you find the taste of tea tree

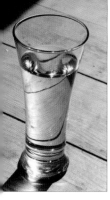

unpleasant, add some honey to the glass. Cider vinegar has therapeutic properties of its own so using cider vinegar with the essential oils will bring added benefits.

Jacuzzis As the water in a Jacuzzi is being constantly circulated, this is an effective way of using essential oils in water; the oils' aroma will be inhaled at the same time. It is important to only use neat oils in the Jacuzzi, as vegetable carrier oils clog up the pump.

Add 6–8 drops of essential oils to the bath once it is filled and ready to be switched on. This number is ideal for a small Jacuzzi, but if the Jacuzzi can take two to three people, add 10 drops.

Saunas Because saunas are so good at eliminating toxins and cleansing the body, the best essential oils to use in them are ones which benefit the respiratory system, such as peppermint, eucalyptus and pine. These are all excellent for clearing catarrh and helping to clear up colds. As they are all strongly antiseptic they are ideal for use in a communal area such as a sauna.

Only 2 drops of essential oil are required in 500 ml of water. Put this on the coals or at the back of the heat source. You need not use much essential oil as the heat of the sauna disperses the aroma very effectively.

VEGETABLE OILS AS A CARRIER

One of the most popular ways of using essential oils, and the main way used by professional aromatherapists, is in massage. As the essential oils are highly concentrated, they are firstly diluted in a vegetable carrier oil. The carrier oil – usually grapeseed or sweet almond – allows for the free movement of the hands during massage.

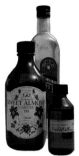

Ideally use cold pressed, top-quality vegetable oils as they contain naturally occurring vitamins and minerals, making them beneficial in their own right. As previously mentioned, baby oil is not suitable. (See p. 142 for more details on carrier oils.)

DILUTION RATE

When massaging an adult, approximately 20 ml of vegetable carrier oil is required; this is equivalent to 4 teaspoons (a plastic medicine spoon = 5 ml). The essential oil should be diluted at $2^{1}/_{2}$%; this equates to 10 drops of essential oil in 20 ml of vegetable oil.

A rate of 2% is used for face massage, i.e. 8 drops of essential oil in 20 ml of carrier oil; while for muscular tension a slightly stronger concentration at 3% is ideal, equivalent to 12 drops in 20 ml of carrier oil.

Some people require a lower dilution, with less essential oil being used. Children need less oil because they are smaller; in pregnant women some of the essential oils will cross the placenta, so less should be used; and in older people, the metabolism is slower and the skin thinner. Anyone over 65 years should have half the normal concentration of essential oils.

Full details of the oil quantities and ratios required for massage are found in the dilution charts on page 33.

BLENDS

A blend of up to three different essential oils can be diluted into the carrier oil, so the total number of drops in a blend come from the three different essential oils. Once essential oils are blended in a carrier oil they should be used within two months; ideally only mix up sufficient for each treatment at a time. Keep the blend in a dark amber glass bottle in the fridge to extend the life of the blend.

OTHER CARRIERS

Base lotions Base lotions or creams are excellent as carriers for applying essential oils to the skin to ease skin disorders such as eczema, psoriasis, burns and sunburns. The advantage of creams and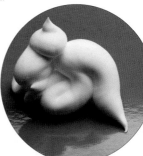

lotions over carrier oils is that they are non-greasy and the cream will be readily absorbed into the skin. Cream is also preferable for burns and sunburn as it is cooling to the skin compared with vegetable oil.

Base lotions and creams are available from aromatherapy suppliers or an unperfumed shop-bought cream can be used; ideally use a natural product.

Similar quantities to carrier oils are used. Most jars are 25 or 50 grams in size so to a 25 gram jar you would add a maximum of 12 drops of essential oil. If it is 50 grams in size, then add 25 drops of essential oil.

When mixing up a facial cream, a 2% dilution should be used, i.e. 8–10 drops in a 25 gram jar.

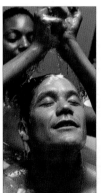

Use a sterilised glass jar and add the essential oils to the cream, using a clean cocktail stick or spoon handle to stir in the oils. With a lotion, shake the jar to mix the essential oils. Label the jar and store in the fridge, where it will last for 2–3 months.

Shampoos Use an unperfumed base shampoo and add essential oils to help conditions like dandruff, eczema, head lice and even alopecia (temporary hair loss).

Put the base shampoo in an amber bottle and add the recommended quantity of essential oil – for example, in a 100 ml bottle add up to 25 drops of essential oil – shake the bottle and use as a normal shampoo.

Bubble baths Add essential oils to an unperfumed bubble-bath base to enjoy all the benefits of the essential oils, knowing they are well dispersed in the bath.

Add the essential oils to the bubble-bath base in a dark-coloured glass bottle at a rate of 25 drops in 100 ml.

Dilution Charts For Essential Oils

ESSENTIAL OILS: DILUTION FOR MASSAGE		
Age group	*Quantity of carrier oil*	*Drops of essential oil*
12–65 years	20 ml	10 drops
6–12 years	20 ml	8 drops
4–6 years	20 ml	5 drops
Elderly	20 ml	5 drops
1–4 years & pregnant women	20 ml	2 drops
Under 1 year	20 ml	1 drop

ESSENTIAL OILS: DILUTION FOR BATHING

Age group	Amount of water	Drops of essential oil
12–65 years	full bath	7–10 drops
4–12 years & elderly	full bath	3–5 drops
Under 4s & pregnant women	full bath	1–2 drops
Under 1 year	full bath	1 drop

ESSENTIAL OILS: DILUTION FOR CREAMS & LOTIONS

Age group	Amount of cream/lotion	Drops of essential oil
12–65 years	50g	25 drops
4–12 years & elderly	50g	12 drops
Under 4s & pregnant women	50g	6 drops
Under 1 year	50g	3 drops

ESSENTIAL OILS:
DILUTION FOR SHAMPOOS & BUBBLE BATHS

Age group	Amount of shampoo/b.bath	Drops of essential oil
12–65 years	100ml	25 drops
4–12 years & elderly	100ml	15 drops
Pregnant women	100ml	8 drops
Under 4s	100ml	3 drops
Under 1 year	100ml	2 drops

ESSENTIAL OILS:
DILUTION FOR BURNERS & COMPRESSES

Burner

6–8 drops of essential oil in water, depending on room size.

4–6 drops if elderly or children are in the room.

Compresses

5–6 drops essential oil in 500ml (1 pint) hot or cold water.

Safety Advice

Although essential oils are 100% natural, they are highly concentrated and therefore need to be diluted. If misused, they can be toxic to the body, so it is important to use the oils correctly.

SKIN PATCH TEST

If your skin is sensitive and you are using an oil for the first time then it is advisable to do a skin or patch test.

Mix one drop of the essential oil in a teaspoon of carrier oil such as grapeseed or sweet almond. Rub some of the mixture on the inside of the wrist or elbow, leave uncovered and unwashed for 24 hours. If there is no sign of redness or itchiness after this time, then it is safe to use.

PHOTOTOXICITY

Most citrus oils, in particular, bergamot, contain a compound called furocoumarin which causes a photo-sensitising effect. This can result in skin pigmentation and sometimes burning if used prior to exposure to sunlight or sunbeds.

Essential oils which are photosensitive are listed on p. 38.

PREGNANCY

One of the main ways essential oils work is by penetrating the skin and so entering the blood stream and lymph system. As the mother's blood supplies the foetus during pregnancy it therefore follows that small percentages of the essential oils used can cross the placenta into the baby. There are a number of safe oils for use during pregnancy which will not harm an unborn baby, but others, such as clary sage, have the ability to stimulate menstruation. These oils are known as emmenogogues and therefore it would be advisable to avoid these during pregnancy.

Oils such as juniper have a stimulating effect on the kidneys while others stimulate the nervous system; these are best avoided in pregnancy. These precautions also apply to mothers who are breastfeeding.

Any essential oils used during pregnancy or while you are breastfeeing should be diluted at lower concentrations. Full details are shown in the charts on p. 33.

BABIES & CHILDREN

Due to their small size and sensitive skin, essential oils should only be used with care and at low dilutions for the under 12s. See the chapter on *Aromatherapy in Pregnancy And For Babies & Children* (p. 181).

On the next page are some key points relating to essential oil safety.

USING ESSENTIAL OILS SAFELY

- Avoid using essential oils about which you can find little or no information
- Do not take the oils internally
- Keep essential oils away from the eyes
- If you do get essential oils in the eyes, wash out immediately with lots of fresh cool water
- Keep essential oils out of the reach of children
- Do not put essential oils neat on the skin; the exceptions are tea tree and lavender
- If epileptic, avoid using rosemary, fennel and sage
- If asthmatic, do not use steam inhalations
- If you are taking homeopathic remedies, avoid the strong-smelling oils such as peppermint – they could weaken the effect of the remedy
- Women who are pregnant should not use basil, juniper, fennel, rosemary, thyme, clary sage, clove, nutmeg, sage, hyssop and wintergreen
- Before going out in sunlight or using a sunbed, avoid using phototoxic citrus oils such as bergamot, grapefruit, lemon, lime, mandarin and orange, although you can use bergamot FCF (see p. 42)
- Some oils irritate sensitive skins, so do a patch test (see p. 36) before using these for the first time: basil, black pepper, cedarwood, geranium, ginger, jasmine, lemon, lemon balm, orange, peppermint, tea tree and ylang ylang

Buying & Storing Essential Oils

These are some pointers on buying and storing oils.

BUYING

- Buy direct from an aromatherapist, mail-order aromatherapy supplier or reputable health-food shop or chemist who can supply information on usage, precautions, etc., when you buy.

- Are the oils diluted? This makes them ready to use, but also expensive to buy. And diluted essential oils cannot be used in a burner.

- The price of each oil in a producer's range should vary due to the cost of production. If you see rose and lavender oil at the same price, it is unlikely that you are buying pure essential oils.

- Look for bottles labelled '100% pure essential oil' – these should be genuine. Bottles of 'aromatherapy' oil could be diluted or a synthetic fragrance. As most essential oils are highly volatile they evaporate quickly

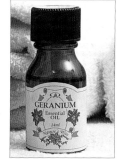

and they are therefore generally kept in sealed dark
brown, blue or green glass bottles. Oils sold in clear
glass or plastic bottles are unlikely to be pure essential oils. Make sure all oils are in labelled bottles.
The bottles should have a dropper cap which allows
you to use one drop of essential oil at a time.

- It is useful to know the Latin names of the oils you
  want so you can make a knowledgeable choice
  when you buy.

STORING

- Keep the oils out of sunlight and direct heat and
  away from food so that they do not pick up smells.
  Ideally store them in a cupboard or drawer, out of
  children's reach. Do not put them on a varnished
  surface as some oils affect wood and varnish.

- Date bottles of citrus oil as they have a life span of
  6–8 months (except bergamot) and can cause skin
  sensitivity if they go rancid. Most others last 3–4
  years and some, like sandalwood, frankincense and
  patchouli, improve with age. Once blended in a
  carrier oil, essential oils have a life span of two
  months so it is best to date home-made blends.

A–Z OF OILS

Each plant's Latin name is included where there are different varieties.

Each oil in this section has advice on its application, but full details on the application of essential oils will be found in *Applying Essential Oils*, p. 19.

PRICE OF ESSENTIAL OILS

In the section that follows there is reference to the price of essential oils; these are categorised in three price bands:

Inexpensive Under £5 for a 10 ml bottle

Medium £5–£10 for a 10 ml bottle

Expensive Over £10 for a 10 ml bottle

Bergamot

Citrus bergamia

This essential oil is very uplifting and a first choice for depression and for giving a psychological boost. The bergamot tree is a native of Bergamo in Italy, hence its name. The oil is expressed from the rind of the bergamot citrus fruit, giving it a fresh, citrus and slightly spicy aroma which is commonly used as an ingredient in eau de Cologne and to flavour Earl Grey tea.

Bergamot is a light greenish-yellow colour and it contains a compound called bergapten. Bergapten can be phototoxic in concentration; in other words, it can cause some sensitivity if you go out in or are exposed to sunlight after using the oil. To overcome this, bergapten- (or furocoumarin-) free bergamot is available; it is commonly known as bergamot FCF. This oil is colourless in comparison.

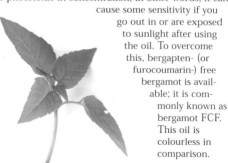

Bergamot plant

PROPERTIES

Bergamot is a must if someone is suffering
from depression or feeling a bit low, as its
fresh uplifting aroma will give a psychological lift, particularly during the 'blues'.
Its invigorating and summery fragrance
is very useful to help people cope with
winter depression in the form of
Seasonal Affected Disorder or SAD.
The psychological boost given by
bergamot will also help those who
are shy or lacking in confidence,
giving them a more positive outlook
on life.

It has antiseptic and astringent properties, which
make bergamot a very good oil for acne sufferers and
those with skin complaints such as eczema and
psoriasis. As it is also uplifting, bergamot will also
help improve the mood of someone depressed because
of acne.

The combination of an antidepressant and an appetite
regulator has made this a useful oil for anyone who is
suffering with anorexia nervosa or from compulsive
eating.

Bergamot has an affinity with the urinary tract and its
antibacterial properties make it ideal to use for cystitis
and urethritis.

APPLICATIONS

BURNERS AND VAPOURISERS

- depression
- feeling fed up
- colds & flu
- SAD
- PMS

DILUTED IN THE BATH OR IN BLENDED OIL

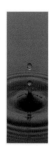

- stress
- tension
- SAD
- PMS
- anxiety
- depression
- feeling fed up
- anorexia nervosa
- any skin condition
- compulsive eating
- postnatal depression
- colds & flu

DILUTED IN A SITZ BATH

- cystitis
- urethritis

BLENDED IN A BASE CREAM

- wounds & cuts
- psoriasis
- oily skin
- scabies
- any skin condition
- eczema
- acne
- cold sores

PRICE RANGE

Medium

BLENDING

Bergamot blends well with many oils and it will bring sharpness to some of the sweetest blends. It works well with camomile, geranium, juniper, lavender, neroli, jasmine and sandalwood.

Blending Note Top

CONTRAINDICATIONS

The main precaution is to avoid going out in sunlight or using a sunbed after application of bergamot. Otherwise, use bergapten-free bergamot, sold as bergamot FCF.

Camomile

Anthemis nobilis or *Chamaemelum nobile*
Matricaria chamomilla or *Matricaria recutica*

This very useful essential oil is renowned for its excellent calming, soothing and healing qualities, both for the mind and body. Its gentle action makes it safe for both adults and children.

Camomile (sometimes spelled chamomile) has a sweet, fruity, apple smell and is pale yellow/green in colour, although German camomile is a deep blue colour.

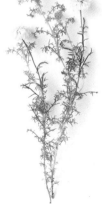

The oil is extracted by steam distillation of the flowering tops of the distinctive, daisy-like camomile plant.

This plant has been used for centuries to scent hair and clothes and for its calming properties. Today, many of us are familiar with camomile tea and the array of beauty products containing camomile.

Roman camomile

Camomile grows throughout Europe and is often spotted growing in fields and hedgerows in Britain.

There are two main types of camomile oil used in aromatherapy:

- the most popular one is Roman or English camomile with the Latin name of *Anthemis nobilis* or *Chamaemelum nobile*. (Latin names are useful to distinguish between different varieties of the same plant, and to make sure that you are buying the correct type of oil.)

- The other camomile you may come across is German or blue camomile (*Matricaria chamomilla* or *Matricaria recutica*).

There is another oil mistakenly called a camomile, but in fact it is not a true camomile. Its name is ormenis flower but is sometimes sold as moroc camomile. It is a fairly new oil and not a lot of research has been carried out on it. It does not contain azulene (see below), but it is generally calming and de-stressing.

PROPERTIES

Both Roman and German camomile contain a naturally occurring substance called azulene and it is this that gives camomile its very calming and soothing property. Azulene is blue in colour and because it is found in such high concentration in German camomile it colours the oil a very distinctive blue. Azulene is anti-inflammatory and therefore both the camomiles are excellent for inflammation of any sort.

Camomile's many other properties include pain relief, particularly with dull aches as opposed to sharp pain. Along with most essential oils it is antiseptic and bactericidal, and so is useful for acne and spots. It can reduce muscle spasm, as experienced in period pain.

Camomile encourages skin growth and so helps to heal scar tissue. Its other qualities enable it to reduce fever and its hypnotic effects will help you sleep.

APPLICATIONS

BURNERS AND VAPOURISERS

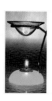

- stress
- depression
- irritability in children
- for psychological effects
- fear
- anxiety & tension

HOT COMPRESS

- period pain
- stomach ache
- inflamed joints
- cystitis
- neuralgia
- arthritis

Cold Compress

- sports injuries
- headaches
- strains & sprains
- arthritis
- acute back pain
- acute neck pain

Blended Oil

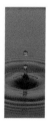

- insomnia
- hayfever
- allergies
- muscle aches
- arthritis
- rheumatic pain
- period pain
- skin complaints
- earache (massage outside of ear)
- stomach ache (massage on tummy)
- toothache/teething (massage on jaw)

Diluted in the Bath

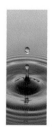

- stress
- anxiety
- tension
- irritability
- PMS
- cystitis
- menopausal symptoms
- skin complaints
- period pain
- insomnia
- muscle aches
- arthritis
- rheumatic pain

DROPS ON A HANDKERCHIEF

- stress
- fear
- irritability
- nausea
- anxiety
- tension
- hayfever
- vomiting

CAMOMILE TEA DRINK

- stomach ache
- insomnia
- period pain
- cystitis
- put camomile tea bags on eyes to relieve sore, itchy and tired eyes

PRICE RANGE

Expensive

BLENDING

Camomile blends well, particularly with bergamot, clary sage, geranium, lavender, neroli, jasmine and rose.

Blending Note Middle

CONTRAINDICATIONS

Camomile is generally very safe, non-toxic and non-irritant. For children and women in early pregnancy, it should be used at half the concentration, i.e. 1%.

Clary Sage

Salvia sclarea

Clary sage is a herb, a member of the sage family, and its main property is to make you feel euphoric! The sage family has many excellent healing properties but unfortunately common sage is not generally safe, so clary sage is the one used in aromatherapy.

The oil is distilled from the flowering tops of clary sage which give oil with a very distinctive and complicated smell, which is nutty, earthy and herbaceous. The aroma is suitable for use by both men and women. Sometimes the smell is not always liked, but it is a very useful oil, so blend it with other oils, particularly citrus oils, to balance the aroma.

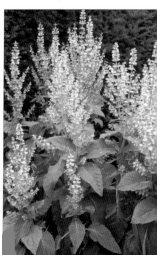

PROPERTIES

Due to its excellent relaxant, antidepressant and euphoric

qualities, this oil is a good choice for stress and depression but it can make you feel drowsy, so it is best used in the evening; do not use it if you are driving or if you may need to drive at some point. It also has the ability to cause hallucinations if you drink alcohol while using this oil. These hallucinations could be pleasant but they could also cause nightmares, so do not use it with alcohol.

Clary sage is a hormone balancer and is therefore beneficial in aiding many gynaecological problems, such as menopause, PMS, menstrual cramps and irregular, heavy or painful periods. It is also used in cases of infertility or impotence.

Clary sage is also a muscle relaxant and so is good for aches and pains, muscle cramp and respiratory problems. It is hypotensive, that is it helps to lower blood pressure, thus benefiting the circulatory system, so use this oil for varicose veins and haemorrhoids.

APPLICATIONS

Burners and Vapourisers

- nervous tension
- depression
- stress
- anxiety
- high blood pressure (h.b.p.)
- insomnia

Hot Compress

- menstrual cramps
- PMS

Blended Oil or Diluted in the Bath

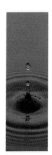

- muscle aches
- frigidity
- migraine
- depression
- anxiety
- h.b.p.
- menstruation problems
- PMS
- asthma
- impotence
- stress
- nervous tension
- insomnia
- irregular periods

Blended in a Cream Base

- haemorrhoids
- varicose veins
- oily & problem skins
- menstrual cramps

Blended in a Base Shampoo

- scalp problems
- oily hair
- hair loss

PRICE RANGE

Medium

BLENDING

Clary sage blends well with many oils, particularly bergamot, frankincense, geranium, jasmine, juniper, lavender, neroli and sandalwood.

Blending Note Top to Middle

CONTRAINDICATIONS

Clary sage is a safe form of sage. It is non-toxic, non-sensitising and non-irritant. **AVOID** during pregnancy due to its emmenagogue (the ability to stimulate menstruation) properties. Do **NOT** use this oil while drinking alcohol as it can induce a narcotic effect.

Eucalyptus

Eucalyptus globulus

This sharp, camphoric, medicinal aroma that is familiar to most people, has been used in remedies for colds and flu for hundreds of years.

The eucalyptus tree is native to Australia and the essential oil used in aromatherapy is extracted by steam distillation from the leaves of the blue gum or globulus variety. It is cheap to extract so this is one of the cheapest essential oils to buy.

The native Aborigines have known the healing properties of eucalyptus for many years and much research has subsequently been carried out on the effectiveness of this oil on the respiratory system. The oil is almost colourless and the odour effect of eucalyptus is enlivening and head-clearing.

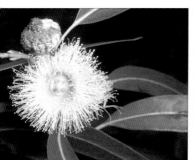

PROPERTIES

It is a must for every home medicine cabinet for its decongestant and antiseptic properties – hence its use for chesty coughs, colds and catarrh. Its head-clearing aroma makes it ideal for treating headaches, migraines, and sinus problems and to help study. It is also beneficial for aches and pains and for arthritis.

Where eucalyptus trees grow it was found they tended to repel mosquitoes, so the oil is commonly used as an insect repellent. As a strong antiseptic it helps kill bacteria in cases of flu, colds and other infections.

The oil has a cooling effect and is useful for fevers and inflammation where there is heat, such as sunburn, arthritis, burns, sprains, chickenpox and measles.

APPLICATIONS

Burners and Vapourisers

- colds & flu
- insect repellent
- coughs
- study purposes
- sinusitis
- headaches
- catarrh

Cold Compress

- burns & sunburn
- sprains
- on the head for headaches, migraines

DROPS ON A HANDKERCHIEF

- blocked sinuses
- colds & flu
- headache
- hayfever

BLENDED OIL OR DILUTED IN THE BATH

- fever
- measles
- arthritis
- aches & pains
- colds & flu
- chickenpox
- rheumatism
- sunburn (cool bath)

STEAM INHALATION

- blocked sinuses
- colds & flu
- catarrh
- hayfever

BLENDED IN A CREAM BASE

- sunburn
- sprains & strains
- measles
- rheumatism
- insect repellent
- burns
- chickenpox
- arthritis
- aches & pains

PRICE RANGE

Inexpensive

BLENDING

Eucalyptus can be quite overpowering but it blends well with lavender, marjoram and rosemary.

Blending Note Top

CONTRAINDICATIONS

 Eucalyptus is non-toxic, non-sensitising and non-irritant but it must be used in low dilutions. **AVOID** in pregnancy and do not use on babies and small children.

Frankincense

Boswellia carteri

The ancient musty aroma of frankincense is reminiscent of the smell of churches and antiquity and it has a history as old as the Bible. The charms and benefits of frankincense were well known by the ancient civilisations of the Greeks, Romans, Persians and Hebrews who used frankincense for both domestic and religious purposes. Frankincense along with myrrh is mentioned in the Bible as a very valuable commodity of that time. Today it is still used as incense in many churches due to its calming and cleansing effect and as an aid to meditation.

The frankincense tree, a native of Oman, and right, the resin from which the oil is extracted

Frankincense is in fact a tree resin, coming from the deserts of Oman, Somalia and Ethiopia and is sometimes known as olibanum. The oil is pale yellow in colour and extracted from the oleo gum resin by steam distillation. This is a fairly expensive process so the oil is relatively dear to buy. It has a musty, warm and balsamic aroma, with a hint of lemon and camphor.

PROPERTIES

This oil has the ability to deepen the breathing, making it an excellent calming and soothing essential oil, beneficial for stress and any breathing problems. Frankincense can help asthma sufferers and anyone with catarrh, bronchitis and coughs.

It has also been found to have anti-inflammatory properties, which can be beneficial for easing the pain of inflamed joints as in arthritis.

As a revitalising tonic for oily and, in particular, mature skins, frankincense is also attributed with the ability to reduce the appearance of wrinkles.

Other benefits include a pronounced soothing effect which can help in times of stress, bereavement and also in women going through the menopause.

It has a very comforting aroma, which helps to give a feeling of security.

APPLICATIONS

BURNERS AND VAPOURISERS

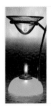

- stress
- insecurity
- bereavement
- bronchitis
- coughs
- catarrh
- laryngitis
- asthma
- nightmares (add a drop to the pillow)

DILUTED IN THE BATH OR IN BLENDED OIL

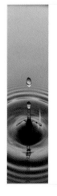

- stress
- insecurity
- menopause
- nightmares
- bereavement
- nervous tension
- PMS
- asthma
- painful periods
- cystitis
- menstruation problems
- uterine bleeding outside of menstruation
- bed wetting in children
- arthritis
- rheumatism
- muscle pain

STEAM VAPORISER

- bronchitis
- catarrh
- coughs
- laryngitis

BLENDED IN A CREAM BASE

- mature skin
- wounds
- acne
- rheumatism
- oily skin
- scars
- arthritis
- muscle aches

PRICE RANGE

Expensive

BLENDING

Frankincense's comforting scent blends very well with all citrus oils including bergamot, geranium, juniper, lavender, neroli, rose and sandalwood.

Blending Note Base

CONTRAINDICATIONS

Frankincense is generally very safe, but as it is an emmenagogue (stimulating menstruation), it is best to **AVOID** in the first 3 months of pregnancy.

Geranium

Pelargonium graveolens

This intensely sweet, floral-smelling oil is a must for women, due to its useful effect on any problems related to hormonal disturbances, such as menopause, menstruation irregularities, cellulite and PMS.

It is extracted from the leaves, stalks and flowers of the rose scented Pelargonium by steam distillation, giving it a greenish colour and making it relatively inexpensive to buy. The aroma is thought to be uplifting and refreshing and its sweet smell is similar to rose. The plant is native to South Africa but is now cultivated worldwide, with most oil being produced in Egypt and Réunion.

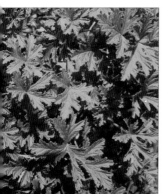

PROPERTIES

Geranium has an overall balancing effect, not only for hormones, but also the skin and the emotions.

Use it for all hormonal irregularities and in skin care its balancing effect makes it suitable for oily, dry and mature skin.

It can be used to treat burns and scalds, and can help soothe other disorders such as shingles, haemorrhoids, ringworm and bruising. The uplifting effect of the oil makes it useful for stress and anxiety, particularly if linked to hormonal irregularities such as menopause and PMS. It is also a diuretic so, again, it is ideal if fluid retention is related to menstruation and PMS. Fluid retention and oedema from other causes will also benefit from geranium, along with cellulitis and cellulite.

Geranium's strong smell can act as an insect repellent, particularly against mosquitos, and it is useful as an aid to combat head lice.

APPLICATIONS

Burners and Vapourisers

- stress
- energising
- mild depression
- PMS
- anxiety & tension
- menopausal symptoms

Diluted in the Bath or Blended Oil

- PMS
- stress
- depression
- anxiety & tension

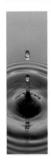

- fluid retention
- oedema
- eczema
- shingles
- cellulitis
- cellulite
- skin complaints
- bruises
- insect repellent
- ringworm
- haemorrhoids
- breast engorgement
- menstrual irregularities
- menopausal symptoms

BLENDED IN A BASE CREAM

- eczema
- shingles
- insect repellent
- ringworm
- all skin types
- haemorrhoids
- burns and scalds
- bruises
- cellulitis and cellulite
- engorgement of the breasts

DILUTED IN A BASE SHAMPOO

- head lice

PRICE RANGE

Medium

BLENDING

Geranium's sweet scent blends very well with bergamot, juniper, lavender, neroli, rose and sandalwood.

Blending Note Middle

CONTRAINDICATIONS

 Although geranium is non-toxic and non-irritant, it can cause sensitivity in some people. Due to its intensely sweet aroma, use it sparingly as it could cause headaches.

Ginger

Zingiber officinale

People have known of the medicinal power of ginger
for centuries and the Greeks and Romans made
extensive use of this very beneficial spice. The plant is
native to Southeast Asia and the rhizomes are used to
produce the spice and essential oil, which is extracted
by steam distillation. The oil is distilled mainly in the
UK and it produces a pale yellow to pale greeny-amber
liquid with a lovely warming, spicy and pungent scent.

PROPERTIES

Ginger's warming aroma makes it ideally suited to all
cases of colds and flu, muscle aches and pains,
arthritis and poor
circulation. Its long
medicinal history includes
its use for digestive upsets
and in particular, nausea
such as morning sickness.
Its stimulating and warm-
ing odour is comforting,
particularly at times of
loneliness or in winter
depression. It has
energising properties,
which make it useful as an
aphrodisiac.

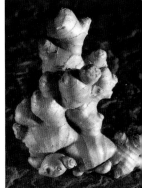

APPLICATIONS

BURNERS AND VAPOURISERS

- catarrh
- nausea
- lethargy
- colds & flu
- feelings of loneliness
- nervous exhaustion
- loss of libido

HOT COMPRESS

- arthritis
- muscle aches
- rheumatism
- digestive upsets

DILUTED IN THE BATH OR BLENDED OIL

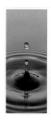

- arthritis
- muscle aches
- rheumatism
- poor circulation
- lethargy
- loss of libido
- colds & flu
- digestive upsets
- nervous exhaustion
- feelings of loneliness

DROPS ON A HANDKERCHIEF

- nausea
- morning sickness
- colds & flu
- indigestion
- travel sickness

BLENDED IN A BASE CREAM

- arthritis
- poor circulation
- muscle aches
- rheumatism

PRICE RANGE

Medium

BLENDING

Ginger has a woody spicy scent which blends well with all the citrus and spicy oils, as well as bergamot, frankincense, neroli, rose, sandalwood and ylang ylang.

Blending Note Middle to Base

CONTRAINDICATIONS

Ginger is non-toxic but can cause skin sensitivity and it is slightly phototoxic. Best to use in low dilutions.

Grapefruit

Citrus paradisi

The zingy, refreshing aroma of this essential oil is reminiscent of summer and so acts as a great psychological lift, particularly in the winter.

The oil is cold-expressed from the peel and is mainly produced in California. It is pale yellow or green in colour with a fresh, sweet citrus fragrance.

Grapefruit does not have a huge range of uses but it is a very valuable oil, mainly for its mood-enhancing aroma, which blends well with most other oils.

PROPERTIES

Like most citrus oils, grapefruit is very uplifting on the spirits so is excellent to use for mild depression and nervous exhaustion. It works as a diuretic so is useful to add to a blend for cellulite. Its astringent qualities can benefit an oily skin or scalp. It is also good for colds, flu and muscle fatigue.

APPLICATIONS

BURNERS AND VAPOURISERS

- mental fatigue
- colds & flu
- mild depression
- nervous exhaustion

DILUTED IN THE BATH OR BLENDED OIL

- cellulite
- colds & flu
- fluid retention
- nervous exhaustion
- muscle fatigue
- mild depression
- obesity

DROPS ON A HANDKERCHIEF

- mild depression
- feeling fed up

PRICE RANGE

Inexpensive

BLENDING

Grapefruit blends well with most citrus and spicy oils

such as bergamot, camomile, geranium, juniper, lavender, neroli, rose, rosemary and tea tree.

Blending Note Top

CONTRAINDICATIONS

Grapefuit is non-toxic, non-irritant, non-sensitising and is phototoxic. Beware: it has a short shelf life of six months, so check the age of the oil when you buy it. Once it begins to oxidise it can cause skin irritation.

Jasmine

Jasminum officinale or *grandiflorum*

Jasmine is one of the most intense floral aromas found in aromatherapy. Its very heady, evocative and warming scent comes from the white flowers of the plant with the smell being at its most intense after dusk. The flowers are generally hand picked at dawn and immediately sent for processing, and with thousands needed to produce a gram of oil, jasmine is one of the most expensive essential oils to buy.

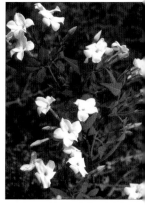

The essential oil is extracted by solvent from the absolute producing oil, deep reddish-brown in colour, which is fairly thick in consistency compared with other oils. It is greatly valued by the perfume industry and most perfumes and some after-shaves contain jasmine for its musky, floral and exotic odour.

Although expensive, very small quantities of the oil are required in order to achieve the benefits and the aroma when applied, will last for hours if not days.

PROPERTIES

In aromatherapy, jasmine is prized mainly for its effect on the emotions. It is a great mood enhancer, energiser and an antidepressant. As an aphrodisiac, it has a reputation for reducing frigidity and impotence.

Jasmine can help in cases of uterine disorders, painful periods and also to relieve labour pains. A useful oil for the respiratory system, jasmine will help ease catarrh, coughs and hoarseness, although there are less expensive oils which can do the job just as well.

Muscle aches and pains can also be relieved with this oil. But the greatest benefit of this oil is with its effect on the nervous system. Jasmine can produce feelings of optimism, confidence and euphoria, particularly when you feel lethargic, indifferent or listless.

APPLICATIONS

Burners and Vapourisers

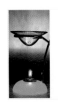

- depression
- menopause
- impotence
- listlessness
- catarrh & other respiratory problems
- PMS
- frigidity
- lethargy

STEAM INHALATION

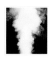

- catarrh
- hoarseness
- coughs
- laryngitis

DILUTED IN THE BATH OR BLENDED OIL

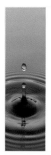

- frigidity
- lethargy
- depression
- greasy skin
- irritated skin
- painful periods
- PMS
- menopause
- impotence
- listlessness
- postnatal depression
- dry skin
- sensitive skin
- labour pains
- uterine disorders
- muscle aches

BLENDED IN A BASE CREAM

- greasy skin
- irritated skin
- dry skin
- sensitive skin

PRICE RANGE

Expensive

BLENDING

Jasmine blends well with bergamot and other citrus oils, clary sage, frankincense, rose and sandalwood.

Blending Note

Middle to Base

CONTRAINDICATIONS

Jasmine is non-toxic and non-sensitising but may slightly irritate the skin of some people. It must **NOT** be used in pregnancy and it is best to avoid using the oil when breast-feeding.

Juniper Berry

Juniperus communis

The fresh, piercing balsamic smell of this oil is indicative of its use as a detoxifying and mind-clearing oil. Juniper has been used for centuries for its antiseptic and diuretic benefits and it was regularly burnt in hospitals and other places where infection was present.

Most people will be familiar with at least one of the main uses of juniper berries nowadays – flavouring gin. The berries are also used to add flavour when cooking.

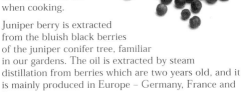

Juniper berry is extracted from the bluish black berries of the juniper conifer tree, familiar in our gardens. The oil is extracted by steam distillation from berries which are two years old, and it is mainly produced in Europe – Germany, France and Italy.

Juniper berry is virtually colourless with a fresh, woody, slightly peppery undertone. Other oils are produced from the needles and wood but these are not suitable for use in aromatherapy.

PROPERTIES

An excellent detoxifier and diuretic, the astringent juniper berry is useful for many disorders including hangovers, skin problems, arthritis, fluid retention, menstrual difficulties and nervous tension. Mentally, it detoxifies and clears the mind, especially when feeling drained or exhausted by other people. It has a great ability to throw off toxins, hence its use with arthritis and gout where it helps eliminate uric acid crystals.

As a detoxifier and astringent, it will help acne and other skin diseases caused by a build up of toxins in the body. The oil's diuretic properties make it useful for fluid retention, cellulite and prostate problems. Juniper berry has a special affinity with the urino-genital tract and it is helpful in cases of cystitis, inflammation of the kidneys and kidney stones, but with these conditions it is important to consult a doctor. It also benefits cases of painful or scant periods.

Juniper berry also has many uses in veterinary care; see *Veterinary Aromatherapy* (see p. 187).

APPLICATIONS

BURNERS AND VAPOURISERS

- hangovers
- colds & flu
- infectious diseases
- for mind-clearing

SITZ BATH

- cystitis
- haemorrhoids

HOT COMPRESS

- cystitis
- painful periods
- arthritis & rheumatism
- aches & pains

BLENDED OIL OR DILUTED IN THE BATH

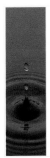

- colds & flu
- cystitis
- painful periods
- hangovers
- mental exhaustion
- all skin conditions
- arthritis & rheumatism
- fluid retention
- cellulite (use stimulating massage)
- aches & pains
- prostate problems
- scant periods
- nervous tension

Blended in a Cream Base

- psoriasis
- acne
- haemorrhoids
- arthritis & gout
- eczema
- oily skin
- cellulite
- aches & pains

PRICE RANGE

Medium to expensive

Blending Note Middle

BLENDING

Juniper berry blends well with bergamot and other citrus oils, clary sage, frankincense, geranium, lavender, rosemary and sandalwood.

CONTRAINDICATIONS

Juniper berry is non-toxic and non-sensitising but may slightly irritate the skin of some individuals. It must **NOT** be used in pregnancy or by people with kidney disease.

French Lavender

Lavandula angustifolia or *Lavandula officinalis*

This is a must for everyone as lavender is the most universal of all the essential oils and it brings benefits to many conditions. If there is only one essential oil at home, then this is the one. It can be safely used on children and can be applied neat in small quantities.

Some of the first research of essential oils was carried out on lavender. It was the French chemist, René Gattefosse, who first discovered the great healing qualities of this oil when he burnt his hand in a laboratory experiment in the 1920s. Dipping the burn in lavender helped to heal the burn without scarring. He subsequently went on to carry out further research on lavender.

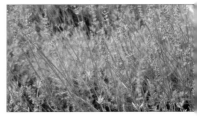

The oil is produced mainly in France and there are various varieties of lavender but the main one to aim for is true or common lavender, called *Lavandula officinalis* or *Lavandula angustifolia*.

The oil is produced from the flowers of the lavender and extracted by steam distillation to produce an oil which is colourless to pale yellow, sweet floral and herbaceous smelling with a woody balsamic undertone.

The vast quantities of lavender oil produced make this an inexpensive oil to purchase.

PROPERTIES

The properties of this oil are vast due to its very complex chemical composition. It can be used for almost anything, from burns, headaches and skin irritations, to PMS and insomnia. But the overall qualities of this oil are calming, soothing and balancing.

It is a gentle oil so it can be safely used on children (more details are given in the section on babies and children, p. 181). It can even be used neat on the skin – one of the few oils that can – in cases of acne, burns and bites.

The first research carried out on this oil showed how very effective it is in treating burns, including sunburn. It will help to heal the skin quickly with little or no scarring.

It is the most effective oil to use for insomnia.

APPLICATIONS

Burners and Vapourisers

- insomnia
- headaches
- PMS
- stress & anxiety
- colds & flu

Steam Inhalation

- colds & flu
- catarrh
- sinusitis

Hot Compress

- period pains
- arthritis
- headaches

Cold Compress

- sprains
- burns and scalds
- insect bites & stings
- headaches
- sunburn

Drops on a Handkerchief

- sudden stress
- hysteria
- panic
- shock
- butterflies in the stomach
- insomnia (drop on pillow)

Blended Oil or Diluted in the Bath

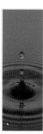

- manic depression
- high blood pressure
- aches & pains
- back ache
- insomnia
- sunburn
- period pain
- stress & anxiety
- PMS
- arthritis
- colds & flu

Blended in base Cream

- sunburn
- scars
- burns
- aches & pains
- acne & spots
- eczema
- cuts & grazes
- arthritis
- insect bites
- scabies

Dabbed neat on skin

- small burns   • acne & spots
- insect bites & stings

PRICE RANGE

Inexpensive

Blending note Middle

BLENDING

Lavender, the universal oil, blends with almost everything, particularly the citrus and floral oils.

CONTRAINDICATIONS

Lavender has no contraindications and
can be used neat in small quantities.
It is also safe to use on children.

Mandarin

Citrus reticulata

This small, sweet citrus fruit was thought to be named after the mandarins of Ancient China after they were offered the fruits as gifts. In common with all citrus oils, mandarin has a lovely, fresh, uplifting citrus smell which will give a psychological boost.

The oil is expressed from the rind of the mandarin and it gives a yellowish-orange colour with a fragrance identical to the smell of the fruit. Originally from China, the fruit is now grown mainly in the Mediterranean.

PROPERTIES

Mandarin is particularly beneficial for the digestive system and because it is so gentle, it is ideal for use on children and the elderly. It has a tonic and stimulant effect on most of the digestive organs and it will help ease a tummy upset in children.

As a relaxant, mandarin is particularly good for treating stress, over-excitement and insomnia.

It is a very refreshing oil to burn

in a vaporiser and, because of its association with Christmas, is good to burn at this time.

Mandarin will encourage skin healing and has been found to be very effective at reducing stretch marks in pregnancy. It can be safely used throughout pregnancy.

APPLICATIONS

BURNERS AND VAPOURISERS

- nervous tension
- over-excitement
- insomnia
- restlessness
- stress, particularly in children, pregnant women and the elderly

BLENDED IN CREAM BASE

- scars
- oily skin
- stretch marks
- acne

BLENDED OIL OR DILUTED IN THE BATH

- nervous tension
- over excitement
- insomnia
- restlessness
- stretch marks (massage the tummy)

- digestive problems (massage the tummy)

- stress, particularly in children, pregnant women and the elderly

PRICE RANGE

Inexpensive

Blending Note Top

BLENDING

Mandarin blends well with bergamot and other citrus oils, camomile, frankincense, geranium, neroli, rose, sandalwood and ylang ylang.

CONTRAINDICATIONS

A very gentle oil, mandarin is non-irritant and non-sensitising, but it can be slightly phototoxic.
It has a short shelf life, so use within 6 to 8 months of purchase.

Sweet Marjoram

Origanum marjorana

Sweet marjoram is a herb found throughout the world and the sedating and calming benefits of this plant have been known for many years.

The essential oil is generally produced in France and other regions of Europe by steam distillation of the flowering tops. This produces a light amber liquid with an aroma which is herby, woody and slightly peppery or nutty. Marjoram is a warming oil and the aroma is suitable for both men and women. Other types of marjoram oil are available but sweet marjoram is the one used in aromatherapy.

PROPERTIES

Marjoram is warming to mind and body and, being anti-spasmodic, will help to ease muscle spasms and period pains. It is de-stressing, calming, good for insomnia and will help lower blood pressure. It is ben-eficial for all muscular aches and pains, rheumatism and arthritis, PMS, and respiratory com-plaints. It is also one of the best oils to use for asthma, bronchitis, coughs and colds.

It has such a sedative effect that it is classed as an anaphrodisiac – i.e. it quells sexual desire.

APPLICATIONS

BURNERS AND VAPOURISERS

• stress	• nervous tension
• insomnia	• PMS
• mental stress	• h.b.p.

BLENDED OIL OR DILUTED IN THE BATH

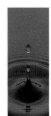

• insomnia	• aches & pains
• h.b.p.	• digestive problems
• arthritis	• rheumatism
• colds	• PMS
• backache	• IBS
• period pains	• mental stress
• anaphrodisiac	• asthma

STEAM INHALATION

• colds
• bronchitis

COLD COMPRESS

- sprains & strains

HOT COMPRESS

- period pains
- migraines
- abdominal pain

BLENDED IN A BASE CREAM

- aches & pains
- arthritis
- chilblains
- bruises

PRICE RANGE

Medium

BLENDING

It blends well with bergamot, camomile, eucalyptus, juniper, lavender, mandarin, rosemary and tea tree.

Blending Note Middle

CONTRAINDICATIONS

 Do **NOT** use in pregnancy.

Neroli

Citrus aurantium var. *amar*

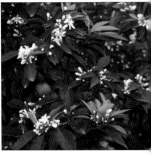

This beautiful-smelling oil comes from the flowers of the bitter-orange tree, also called the Seville orange. It is thought a 17th-century princess of Neroli gave her name to the oil, as she used it to scent her gloves. Neroli has long been used as a perfume, most famously in the eau de Cologne 4711, along with orange, bergamot and rosemary oils.

It is one of the most expensive oils, as it takes a tonne of hand-picked flowers to produce one litre of essential oil. The oil is extracted by steam distillation and is coloured a pale yellow, which darkens with age. The tree is native to the Far East, but the oil is now produced mainly in Italy, Egypt and France. The by-product of the distillation of neroli is orange flower water.

The aroma of neroli oil is fresh and powerful yet light, with a sharp, flowery undertone. Two other essential oils also come from this tree: petitgrain from the twigs and leaves, and bitter orange oil from the fruit's rind. Both of these oils are much less expensive than neroli.

PROPERTIES

Neroli's main effects lie in its calming ability on the emotions and nervous system. It is the first choice for shock and hysteria and is also helpful for stress-related high blood pressure, palpitations and any form of nervous anxiety. It is an emotionally supportive oil and benefits anyone who feels depressed and a loss of hope. Neroli is useful for the emotional symptoms of PMS, menopause and postnatal depression.

Physically, neroli's calming properties are ideal for digestive upsets such as diarrhoea, particularly due to nervous tension. It has long been used in skincare and can benefit most skin types. Its rejuvenative properties make it particularly beneficial for mature and sensitive skins, stretch marks and in helping to heal scars.

APPLICATIONS

BURNERS AND VAPOURISERS

- anxiety
- PMS
- depression
- h.b.p.

BLENDED IN A BASE CREAM

- stretch marks
- thread veins
- mature & sensitive skins
- scars
- wrinkles

BLENDED OIL OR DILUTED IN THE BATH

- diarrhoea
- muscle spasm
- anxiety
- PMS
- colic
- palpitations
- depression
- h.b.p.

DROPS ON A HANDKERCHIEF

- sudden shock
- palpitations
- depression
- hysteria
- anxiety
- h.b.p.

PRICE RANGE

Expensive

BLENDING

Neroli oil blends with almost everything, particularly camomile, geranium, clary sage, jasmine, lavender, rose and ylang ylang.

Blending Note Middle to Base

CONTRAINDICATIONS

Neroli has no contraindications.

Peppermint

Mentha piperita

The fresh and stimulating aroma of this oil is familiar to all of us, as the oil has been used as a flavouring agent in toothpaste and confectionery for many years.

The Ancient Greeks and possibly the Egyptians used peppermint leaves to help digestion and there is evidence that they laid the leaves on the ground to help reduce the spread of disease and to dispel foul smells. The oil still has many uses today: as well as in aromatherapy, peppermint is used as a flavouring for cordials, toothpaste, etc. and it is used in liqueurs such as Crème de Menthe, Chartreuse and Benedictine.

There are many types of mint, but peppermint is especially beneficial as it contains large quantities of menthol, source of its cooling, pain-relieving properties. The essential oil is produced mainly in the USA, China and Japan, by steam distillation of the flowering tops, giving an oil which is colourless to pale yellow. Peppermint oil has a very distinctive aroma, which is piercing fresh, minty and very head-clearing.

PROPERTIES

Peppermint is excellent for all digestive disorders, including nausea, indigestion, heartburn, stomach-ache and flatulence. The best way to use it is diluted and massaged onto the tummy. It has anti-inflammatory properties and is good for Irritable Bowel Syndrome (IBS); peppermint capsules are also available which can be taken internally to relieve the symptoms of IBS.

Peppermint is very refreshing and cooling and is therefore beneficial for fevers and sunburn. Its head-clearing aroma is excellent for studying, relieving headaches and as a room freshener, although you should not use at night, as it may keep you awake. It also helps with colds, flu and blocked sinuses.

Vermin such as ants, cockroaches and mice do not like this aroma, so you can sprinkle it on their runs as an environmentally friendly way of deterring them.

APPLICATIONS

Burners and Vapourisers

- sinusitis
- catarrh
- room freshener
- headaches
- as an aid to study & concentration
- colds & flu
- mental fatigue
- migraines

COLD COMPRESS

- migraines
- bruises
- muscle pain & swelling
- sunburn (use with lavender)
- headaches

DROPS ON A HANDKERCHIEF

- headaches
- indigestion
- shock
- nausea
- to aid study & concentration
- migraines
- sinusitis
- fainting
- vertigo

BLENDED OIL OR DILUTED IN THE BATH

- fever (cool bath)
- sunburn (cool bath)
- IBS
- any digestive disorder
- muscle aches & pains

STEAM INHALATION

- sinusitis
- colds & flu
- catarrh

BLENDED IN A CREAM BASE

- sprains & strains
- sunburn
- IBS (rub on tummy)
- aches & pains
- headaches & migraines (rub on temples)
- toothache (rub on jaw)

DRINK PEPPERMINT TEA

- indigestion
- stomach upset
- nausea
- heartburn
- flatulence
- colic
- headaches
- IBS
- after dinner to aid digestion

PRICE RANGE

Inexpensive

BLENDING

Peppermint's very distinctive smell makes it difficult
to blend, but in small quantities it goes well with clary
sage, eucalyptus, marjoram, lavender, rosemary and
tea tree.

Blending Note Top

CONTRAINDICATIONS

Peppermint is very powerful, so use it in
low dilutions and be very careful using
it on skin as irritation can result. **AVOID**
in pregnancy and do not use on babies
or young children, i.e. under 3 years. Do
not use if using homeopathy as it can
hinder the effects.

Rose

Rosa centifolia or Rosa damascena

Rose is commonly known as the queen of the essential oils as it was one of the first oils to be distilled back in the 10th century by the Persian physician, Avicenna.

The rose's very special qualities have been known for centuries and it has a history as a symbol of love and beauty. Rose essential oil is one of the most expensive, as its takes tonnes of petals to produce a small quantity of the oil – but only small amounts of the oil need to be used because of its powerful, flowery scent.

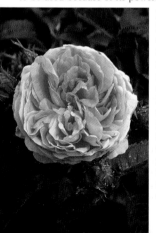

Rose otto is produced by steam distillation mainly in Morocco, the centre of cultivation of roses for oil production; this is the oil generally preferred for aromatherapy and rose water is a by-product of its distillation. Another essential oil is produced, known as rose absolute, which is obtained by solvent extraction of the fresh petals. Larger quantities of rose absolute are produced, mainly for the perfume industry, so it is generally cheaper to buy.

Rose otto is almost colourless with a sweet, mellow and slightly spicy, flowery scent, which can be quite heady; while rose absolute is deep yellow to red in colour with a rich, sweet, mellow flowery scent.

There are two species of rose used in essential oil production: Damask Rose (*Rosa damascena*), which is deep pink in colour and grown mainly in Bulgaria and Turkey; and Cabbage Rose (*Rosa centifolia*), pale pink and grown mainly in Morocco, Tunisia and France.

PROPERTIES

Rose has a special affinity with women and especially with the womb. It is a very beneficial oil to use for reproductive complaints, including PMS, menopause, lack of muscle tone in the womb, and helping regulate the menstrual cycle, making it useful in cases of infertility. It is a gentle antidepressant, particularly if associated with sexual problems or reproduction, and is helpful in cases of postnatal depression. It is also an aphrodisiac and will help in cases of frigidity and male impotence and all cases of stress and nervous tension.

Rose has a long history of use in skin care: most people will be familiar with rose water as a skin toner. Rose will benefit all skin types, particularly mature, dry or sensitive skins and it will help to reduce thread veins on the cheeks if used over a long period.

Rose is beneficial for other complaints such as hayfever, coughs, catarrh and poor circulation, but there are other less expensive alternatives for these conditions so rose is generally used in aromatherapy purely for its psychological effects and for its great benefit to the female reproductive system.

APPLICATIONS

BURNERS AND VAPOURISERS

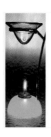

- stress
- bereavement
- nervous tension
- relationship breakdown
- postnatal depression
- anxiety
- grief

BLENDED IN A BASE CREAM

- dry skins
- mature skins
- sensitive skins
- thread veins

BLENDED OIL OR DILUTED IN THE BATH

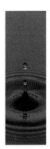

- PMS
- infertility
- frigidity
- stress
- nervous tension
- postnatal depression
- relationship breakdown
- grief
- irregular periods
- prolapsed womb
- impotence
- anxiety
- bereavement

PRICE RANGE

Expensive

BLENDING

Rose oil blends with many oils, including bergamot, camomile, clary sage, geranium, jasmine, lavender, neroli and sandalwood.

Blending Note Middle to Base

CONTRAINDICATIONS

Rose has no contraindications and is safe to use. As it is a mild emmenagogue (it stimulates menstruation), it is best avoided in the first 3 months of pregnancy.

Rosemary

Rosamarinus officinalis

This stimulating herb has long been used in medicine and for culinary purposes. Rosemary has always been known to improve the memory and the Greeks would wear a garland of rosemary around their heads to increase concentration during study. Rosemary is often added to food, particularly to combat fatty foods such as lamb, and in the past its strong bactericidal properties saw it used to prevent decay in uncooked meat.

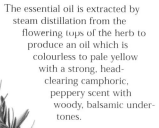

The essential oil is extracted by steam distillation from the flowering tops of the herb to produce an oil which is colourless to pale yellow with a strong, head-clearing camphoric, peppery scent with woody, balsamic undertones.

Rosemary for essential oil production is mainly grown in France, Spain and Tunisia, although it is found all over the world. The oil is inexpensive and is an ingredient of Eau de Cologne. Napoleon was a great advocate of rosemary cologne, using it for concentration when planning military manoeuvres.

PROPERTIES

Rosemary is used for a wide range of complaints, from respiratory and circulatory disorders to muscular aches and pains and hair care. It is very stimulating both on the mind and body and it is especially useful for study and to improve concentration. The stimulating properties will benefit poor circulation, low blood pressure, fluid retention and cellulite.

Rosemary is also analgesic (pain relieving), helping to ease arthritis, rheumatism, all aches and pains, neuralgia and painful periods. It is particularly useful for sports people, for massage both before and after exercise.

Its stimulating properties aid the digestive system in cases of constipation, IBS, stomach pains and flatulence, and it acts as a tonic for the liver as well as the heart. Rosemary is strongly antiseptic and antibacterial and will benefit the respiratory system in cases of asthma, bronchitis, catarrh and coughs.

Rosemary will help energise if feeling tired or mentally exhausted, but do not use it in the evening otherwise it will keep you awake.

As a stimulant to blood circulation, rosemary is beneficial in cases of temporary hair loss (alopecia). Wash hair with rosemary to help clear dandruff and use it on dark and oily hair to add lustre. Head lice can be controlled with rosemary, particularly if used with tea tree.

APPLICATIONS

BURNERS AND VAPOURISERS

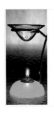

- coughs
- colds & flu
- sinusitis
- room freshener
- headaches
- migraines
- to aid study & concentration
- to energise the mind

STEAM INHALATION

- coughs
- colds & flu
- sinusitis
- catarrh
- bronchitis

COLD COMPRESS

- sprains & strains
- headaches
- migraines

BLENDED OIL OR DILUTED IN THE BATH

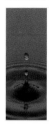

- arthritis
- aches & pains
- backache
- poor circulation
- cellulite
- colds & flu
- neuralgia

- rheumatism
- sprains & strains
- low blood pressure
- low energy
- fluid retention
- general infection
- painful periods

BLENDED IN A SHAMPOO BASE

- scabies
- dandruff

- head lice
- alopecia

PRICE RANGE

Inexpensive

BLENDING

Rosemary oil blends with citrus oils, frankincense, lavender and peppermint.

Blending Note Middle

CONTRAINDICATIONS

Rosemary must **NOT** be used if you are pregnant or suffer epilepsy or high blood pressure.

Sandalwood

Santalum album

The heady, smooth, sweet, mellow and woody scent of this essential oil has been prized for many years for its long-lasting, sensual aroma and excellent skincare properties. It has been used in the East for thousands of years as an incense, a perfume and for embalming.

The oil comes from a small, tropical, parasitic evergreen that takes 20 years to mature sufficiently to produce the oil. Native to southern Asia, most of the world's sandalwood supply now comes from Mysore

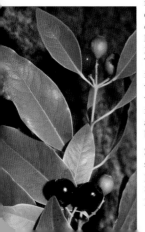

in India. The oil is extracted by steam distillation from the dried heartwood and roots of 20- to 50-year-old trees. The oil is a thick, yellowish-brown sticky liquid with a sweet balsamic and woody smell and the scent improves with age. The aroma is popular with both men and women.

Sandalwood is still used in skin preparations, incense, perfumes and after-shaves, mainly for its long-lasting properties.

PROPERTIES

This is a deeply relaxing, sensual and soothing oil with many beneficial properties: it is anti-inflammatory, antibacterial, a respiratory and urinary antiseptic, fever-reducing, a sedative and an antidepressant. It is also an effective aphrodisiac.

Sandalwood is one of the best choices for problems with the respiratory system, particularly in cases of dry, persistent and irritating coughs when it is best applied diluted, to the outside of the chest and throat.

APPLICATIONS

BURNERS AND VAPOURISERS

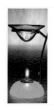

- bronchitis
- coughs
- sore throat
- insomnia
- nervous tension
- catarrh
- laryngitis
- depression
- stress
- PMS

STEAM INHALATIONS

- bronchitis
- coughs
- sore throat
- catarrh
- laryngitis

BLENDED OIL OR DILUTED IN THE BATH

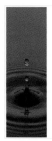

- bronchitis
- catarrh
- coughs
- laryngitis
- sore throat (massage on throat)
- diarrhoea
- nausea
- depression
- insomnia
- stress
- nervous tension
- cystitis (massage on tummy)
- PMS

BLENDED IN A BASE CREAM

- mature skin
- dry skin
- acne
- inflamed skin
- eczema
- psoriasis
- shaving rashes
- chapped & cracked skin

PRICE RANGE

Expensive

BLENDING

Sandalwood oil blends well with many others, including bergamot, frankincense, jasmine, juniper berry, geranium, lavender, rose and ylang ylang.

Blending Note Base

CONTRAINDICATIONS

 Sandalwood has no contraindications and is very safe to use. It can be safely used in pregnancy.

Tea Tree

Melaleuca alternifolia

A lot of research has been carried out on this very powerful oil for its antibacterial, antifungal and antiviral properties. Although difficult to use in a blend for massage due to its antiseptic, clinical smell, tea tree is a must for the first-aid kit.

Sometimes known as ti tree, the plant is native to New South Wales. It is part of the melaleuca family which yields two other essential oils – niaouli and cajeput, both also antiseptic. This tree's properties have been known to native Aborigines for many years, with its leaves used as poultices, infusions and ointments for infected wounds, inhalations and respiratory complaints.

Tea tree is a small tree with short, needle leaves and bottlebrush-like yellowy flowers. The essential oil is extracted from the leaves and twigs by steam distillation, giving a pale yellow liquid. The aroma is powerfully strong with a medicinal smell similar to juniper or eucalyptus.

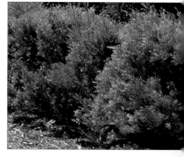

PROPERTIES

It is a very strong natural antiseptic, antibiotic, antiviral and antifungal, so it is useful for many first-aid situations. It can be used neat and is safe for use on children. Tea tree is excellent for spots, cuts, bites, acne, cystitis and thrush, dandruff, warts, colds, flu, and sore throats. It will generally stimulate the immune system, so it is good to use when people around you have colds or flu.

The antifungal properties make it useful against ringworm and athlete's foot, warts, dandruff, cradle cap and candida albicans. And as an excellent immune-system stimulant, tea tree has recently been researched to test its effectiveness against the HIV virus.

APPLICATIONS

BURNERS AND VAPOURISERS

- disinfect a room
- colds & flu

COLD COMPRESS

- sunburn   • burns
- wounds
- insect bites & stings

BLENDED OIL OR DILUTED IN THE BATH

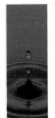

- insect bites & stings
- sunburn
- colds & flu
- cystitis
- thrush
- athlete's foot
- foot infections
- ringworm
- burns
- wounds
- candida albicans
- glandular fever
- chicken pox

BLENDED IN A SHAMPOO BASE

- dandruff
- cradle cap
- chicken pox
- itchy scalp
- any fungal infections

BLENDED IN A CREAM BASE

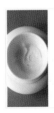

- acne
- sunburn
- athlete's foot
- foot infections
- cold sores
- ringworm
- burns
- wounds
- nappy rash
- chicken pox
- insect bites & stings

As A Gargle

- sore throats
- bad breath
- mouth ulcers
- colds & flu

Dabbed on neat

- acne
- warts & veruccae
- cuts & grazes
- insect bites
- cold sores

In a Sitz Bath

- cystitis
- thrush

PRICE RANGE

Inexpensive

BLENDING

Tea tree blends well with clary sage, eucalyptus, geranium, lavender, marjoram and rosemary.

Blending Note Top

CONTRAINDICATIONS

Tea tree has no contraindications. It can irritate sensitive skins, so ideally dilute it in these cases. It can be used neat in small quantities. It is safe to use on children.

Ylang Ylang

Cananga odorata var. *genuina*

This exotic oil with its heady fragrance evokes memories of its tropical Asian origins: most of the oil is produced in the Seychelles, Madagascar and Réunion.

Ylang ylang (pronounced e-lang e-lang) is a pale yellow oil, extracted from the yellow blooms of this tall tropical tree. Its heavy, sweet, exotic and sometimes overpowering scent is extensively used in perfumes. In Victorian times the oil was widely used in a hair preparation called macassar oil, as a hair tonic.

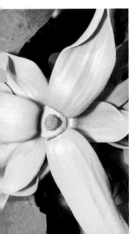

The oil is extracted from the flowers by steam distillation and four distillations are taken. The first distillation known as 'extra', is the top grade and the best one to use in aromatherapy. The successive ones are called first, second and third grade.

PROPERTIES

Ylang ylang's main property is one of relaxation. Its aroma is similar to jasmine but it is not so expensive.

Its relaxing qualities make it is very useful for those who are stressed, anxious or tense and it can even help to lower blood pressure. Ylang ylang is beneficial for anyone who gets palpitations when stressed, as it helps slow down rapid breathing and over-rapid heart rate. It has excellent qualities for skin and hair care.

The oil's warming, intoxicating aroma is said to be an aphrodisiac and, combined with its antidepressant effects, it can help in cases of sexual inadequacy.

APPLICATIONS

BURNERS AND VAPOURISERS

- insomnia
- h.b.p.
- depression
- PMS
- relaxation & stress relief

A DROP ON A HANDKERCHIEF

- palpitations
- panic attacks
- over-rapid breathing
- over-rapid heartbeat

BLENDED IN A BASE CREAM

- dry or oily skin
- acne

Diluted in the Bath or as a Blended Oil

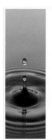

- h.b.p.
- anxiety & tension
- stress
- fear
- depression
- frigidity
- impotence
- PMS
- palpitations
- panic attacks
- over-rapid breathing
- over-rapid heartbeat
- insomnia

PRICE RANGE

Medium

Blending Note Middle to Base

BLENDING

Ylang ylang's beautiful perfume blends well with bergamot, clary sage, frankincense, jasmine, geranium, grapefruit, lavender, neroli and rose.

CONTRAINDICATIONS

Ylang ylang has no major contraindications although it can irritate sensitive skins. Due to its very heady scent it is best to use only in small quantities as it can cause headaches and nausea.

USING ESSENTIAL OILS AT HOME

Essential oils have many uses, particularly in the home. This section suggests uses and quick and easy recipies. For more details of how to use the oils, see the section on *Applying Essential Oils* (p. 19) and adjust the quantity of oils according to age group – see *Dilution Charts for Essential Oils*, pp. 33–35.

MORNING SHOWER OR BATH

- **Wake up sleepy head!** 3 drops of bergamot; 3 drops of rosemary; 4 drops of grapefruit

- **Cleansing wash** ideal for oily or blemished skin and for men: 2 drops of tea tree; 2 drops of rosemary; 6 drops of grapefruit

- **Citrus zing** very refreshing blend for the morning: 4 drops of mandarin; 4 drops of grapefruit; 2 drops of neroli

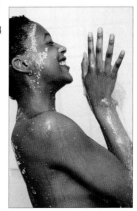

- **Breathe easy** this blend helps clear a blocked nose, ready to face the day: 6 drops of eucalyptus; 2 drops of clary sage; 2 drops of frankincense

HOUSEWORK WITH ESSENTIAL OILS

Their antibacterial properties make essential oils useful to clean the house as well as environmentally safer than many chemicals.

- **Disinfectant spray** use to clean work surfaces and to disinfect where children play: 150 ml of white vinegar; 100 ml of water; 20 drops of tea tree. Put the essential oils in white vinegar and water in a plant spray bottle, shake and then spray.

- **Freshen up the vacuum cleaner** freshen the room as you clean: put a pad of cotton wool with 8 drops of essential oil in the bag of your vacuum cleaner or put 8 drops directly on a felt filter.
Use 6 drops of eucalyptus with 2 drops of sandalwood or alternatively use 8 drops of cedarwood.

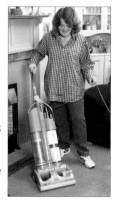

- **Carpet aromatherapy** use essential oils to inject some life back into your carpet:

put bicarbonate of soda, Fullers earth or an unperfumed talcum powder into a plastic bag, add 30 drops of essential oil, close the bag and shake. Leave a for few hours for the powder to absorb the essential oils then sprinkle on the carpet, wait half an hour and then vacuum.

- **Add a zing to your washing** put 4 drops of bergamot or any citrus essential oil in the fabric conditioner drawer of the washing machine to add a refreshing aroma to your washing.

ROOM FRESHENERS

Using a plant spray bottle, add 10 drops of essential oils to 250 ml of water, shake then spray to clear stuffy or smoky rooms or disguise cooking smells. You can also use these blends in a burner or diffuser.

- **Blitz cooking smells** 2 drops of peppermint; 4 drops of lavender; 4 drops of clary sage
- **Clear away cigarette smoke** 2 drops of rosemary; 3 drops of tea tree; 5 drops of eucalyptus

MOOD ENHANCING BLENDS

Use these blends in a burner, plant spray or vaporiser to enhance a room's ambience.

- **Ladies' coffee morning** refreshing blend for the morning coffee and biscuit break: 5 drops of mandarin; 3 drops of bergamot; 2 drops of geranium

- **Dinner party relaxer** great to burn to create a relaxed atmosphere for your dinner party guests, this contains both feminine and masculine scents: 6 drops of bergamot; 2 drops of geranium; 2 drops of sandalwood

- **Seductive nights** blend to relax to in the evening, excellent for the bedroom! 2 drops of ylang ylang; 2 drops of rose; 6 drops of grapefruit

- **Christmas warmer** warming blend to use on cold winter nights: 7 drops of mandarin; 2 drops of frankincense; 1 drop of ginger

HOME-MADE CANDLES

These are easy to make.

1 Use a very fat candle and select your favourite essential oils – perhaps a blend suggested above.

2 Light the candle, leave for a few minutes to let the wax melt around the wick then blow out.

3 Add your chosen oils to the melted wax, then relight.

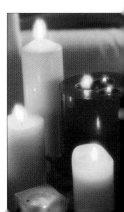

The effect lasts for about 30 minutes. You will need to repeat the process if you want to prolong the aroma.

SKIN CARE WITH AROMATHERAPY

Essential oils come into their own with beauty and hair care, bringing many benefits to the health and condition of the hair, skin and body.

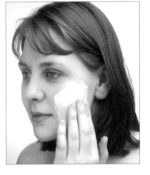

FACIAL CREAMS

Use a base lotion or cream for your blends or make your own 100% natural creams, as shown here.

- **100% natural home-made cream** a firm-set cream ideal for use as a cleansing cream, light moisturiser or hand cream: 40 ml of sweet almond oil; 10 g of beeswax; 40 ml of rosewater (or orange water)
- **Cocoa butter cream** a much richer face cream: 50 ml of sweet almond oil; 35 g of cocoa butter; 10 g of beeswax; 45 ml of rosewater

Makes approximately three 50 gram jars. Add a maximum total of 20 drops of essential oil to a 50 gram jar.

1 Cut up the beeswax and cocoa butter very finely

and melt in a bowl over hot water (bain marie).

2 Add the warmed base oil very slowly.

3 Warm the rosewater and add it very slowly, whisking all the time (like making mayonnaise), until all the rosewater is used up.

4 Pour into sterilised dark-coloured jars and then put in the fridge. The cream will last there for several months.

5 When you need another jar, re-melt the cream in a bain marie. Do not be tempted to warm the cream in a microwave as a big mess will result!

6 Add your chosen essential oils as required, stirring them into the melted cream using a cocktail stick.

BLENDS FOR FACIAL CREAMS

All the specific recipes that follow are for a 25 gram jar, using a total of 8 drops of essential oil.

- **Regenerate dehydrated skin** very moisturising for dry or dehydrated skin. Use a base cream or the rich home-made cream (p. 123) for the base: 3 drops of camomile; 3 drops of neroli; 2 drops of rose

- **Rejuvenate mature skin** help reduce the wrinkles with this blend. Use a base cream or the rich home-made cream (p. 123) for the base: 4 drops of frankincense; 2 drops of neroli; 2 drops of rose

- **Neutralise oil** perfect for oily skin. Use base lotion:

4 drops of bergamot; 2 drops of juniper; 2 drops of frankincense

- **Calm down spots** for acne-prone skin with an astringent, masculine aroma ideal for teenage boys. Use base lotion or jojoba oil as the carrier: 3 drops of tea tree; 3 drops of rosemary; 2 drops of frankincense

PERFUMES

- **Perfume** dilute your favourite essential oils in jojoba oil, i.e. rose or jasmine, or use the blend below: 2 drops of jasmine; 6 drops of ylang ylang; in 10 ml of jojoba oil

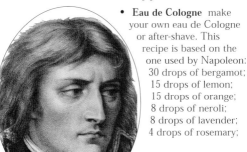

- **Eau de Cologne** make your own eau de Cologne or after-shave. This recipe is based on the one used by Napoleon: 30 drops of bergamot; 15 drops of lemon; 15 drops of orange; 8 drops of neroli; 8 drops of lavender; 4 drops of rosemary;

Napoleon Bonaparte: his eau de Cologne inspired the one given above

in 100 ml of distilled water, perfume grade-alcohol
or vodka).

1 Put all the essential oils into a dark-coloured bottle,
add the distilled water and shake. (Perfume-grade
ethyl alcohol or vodka will make the blend last
longer.)

2 Leave the bottle in a cool dark place for a few days
or weeks to mature, before using.

• **After-shave** prepare in the same way as eau de
Cologne: 8 drops of bergamot; 6 drops of juniper; 6
drops of lavender; 3 drops of sandalwood; 3 drops
of frankincense; in 50 ml of witch hazel, perfume-
grade alcohol or vodka.

HAIR CARE WITH AROMATHERAPY

SHAMPOO

Add 25 drops of your chosen essential oils to a base
shampoo and keep in a dark-coloured bottle.

• **Blitz dandruff** 15 drops of tea tree; 10 drops of
rosemary

• **Restore hair** to help reduce alopecia: 5 drops of
clary sage; 5 drops of lavender; 15 drops of rosemary

• **Blend for greasy hair** 15 drops of grapefruit; 5
drops of juniper; 5 drops of rosemary

A GOOD NIGHT'S SLEEP WITH AROMATHERAPY

Bath Blends

For use of essential oils in the bath, see Applying Essential Oils on p. 25.

- **Sweet dreams** add these oils to a full bath, lie back and start dreaming: 4 drops of clary sage; 2 drops of neroli; 2 drops of sandalwood

- **Unknot those aching muscles** 2 drops of camomile; 5 drops of lavender; 3 drops of marjoram

- **Sleep tight** if you have difficulty getting to sleep, the simple way to help is to put a couple of drops of lavender (or camomile, if you prefer) on your pillow before you lie down, one at either corner. Keep

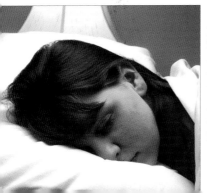

the bottle by the bed so that if you wake up in the night you can add more drops. (Do not use dark-colour oils on light-coloured bedding.)

AROMATHERAPY AT WORK

Don't forget to take your essential oils to work where they can help to ease the stresses of your day.

IN YOUR CAR

Oils can be used in the car to help de-stress your journey, or perhaps you need to wake up on your journey to work?

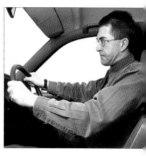

- **Stressful journey?** put 3 to 4 drops of peppermint or eucalyptus essential oil on a tissue and put this by the car's heater outlet to help fragrance the interior; alternatively sprinkle a few drops of essential oil on the carpets. Be wary of putting dark-coloured oils on light-coloured carpets.

BLENDS FOR THE OFFICE

When selecting a blend, be aware of any contraindications of colleagues in the same room; for example anyone who is pregnant or suffering from high blood pressure (see *Safety Advice,* p. 36). In an office, it is safest to use an electric diffuser or vaporiser.

- **Cold buster** Essential when colleagues are suffering with colds or flu, as it helps reduce the spread of infection: 4 drops of eucalyptus; 2 drops of tea tree; 2 drops of rosemary

- **Brain stimulant** When you need extra brain power to tackle that important meeting or challenging piece of work: 2 drops of peppermint; 3 drops of rosemary; 3 drops of eucalyptus

- **PMS week** If you or your colleagues are suffering the symptoms of PMS, try this blend at work to ease your day: 2 drops of bergamot; 2 drops of clary sage; 3 drops of geranium; 1 drop of rose or neroli

- **Energising blend** If your energy flags at the end of the day, use this blend to re-energise you: 4 drops of bergamot; 4 drops of grapefruit; 2 drops of juniper

- **Office tension?** when there is tension in the office, this blend will help to soothe the atmosphere: 2 drops of marjoram; 1 drop of clary sage; 3 drops of bergamot; 3 drops of grapefruit

TISSUE POWER

A few drops of an essential oil on a tissue or hankie can bring many benefits during the day. If you have sensitive skin, be careful not to let the oils come into direct contact with your skin.

- **Colds, blocked sinuses or a headache?** Put 2 to 3 drops of eucalyptus or 1 drop of peppermint on a tissue and tuck inside your shirt, blouse or bra. The warmth of your body will disperse the aromas, helping to clear your head.

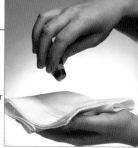

- **Nerve-racking situation?** Before a presentation, examination or perhaps a dental visit, use lavender oil to calm your nerves. Put 3 to 4 drops of lavender on a tissue and use as above.

- **Need cheering up?** Put 3 to 4 drops of bergamot or grapefruit on a tissue and use as above.

OFFICE MASSAGE

If you suffer tension headaches at work then a few simple massage techniques using lavender oil can help ease them.

- **Temple rub** Put a drop of lavender on your fingers and rub this into your temples (the slight indentation at the side of the head, in line with the eyebrows). Gently massage the temples in an anti-clockwise direction using your fingertips. This can bring instant relief.

- **Temple squeeze** With a drop of lavender oil on your palms, try another technique for headache relief.

Place your hands either side of the head with your palms on your temples and fingertips pointing towards the ceiling. Make big circular moves with the heels

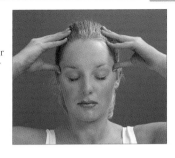

of the hands, then squeeze your head between your hands as hard as possible.
Maintaining the pressure, slowly lift your hands upwards and take your fingers though your hair, gently pulling upwards.

This wonderful releasing technique feels as though your headache is being taken up and away from your head.

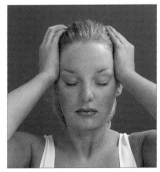

• **Eye strain**
  If you
  spend long
  hours in
  front of a
  computer,
  you may
  find you
  suffer with
  eye strain.
  Have regu-
  lar eye tests
  to make
  sure your
  sight is not
  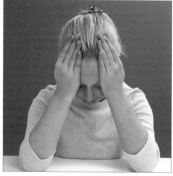
  suffering and take regular screen breaks.
  Use this technique to help ease any eye strain.
  Rest your elbows on the desk and place your hands
  over your shut eyes, with your palms cupped over
  your eye sockets. Keep this position for a few minutes and the warmth of your palms will soothe sore
  and tired eyes.

BLENDING

Following on from the application and use of essential oils, the next stage is to try some creative blending.

Early aromatherapy research discovered that essential oils are therapeutically more effective if used in a blend of three or four oils rather than using the oils on their own. Blended oils help to enhance one another's properties, so the overall effect is greater than the sum of the individual parts. Using this knowledge, most aromatherapists will use a mixture of oils when preparing blends for clients. This also lets the aromatherapist work on more than one complaint at a time, taking into account all the emotional and physical needs of the client.

When mixing up a blend of essential oils, various factors are taken into account:

- The present health of the individual should be noted to help any emotional and physical problems.

- It is important that oils are used which blend well together and produce a favourable aroma.

- Other things taken into consideration include whether the individual needs an uplifting or stimulating blend: perhaps they are driving or going out afterwards; or perhaps it is evening and they would benefit from a relaxing blend.

One of the most important aspects of the blend is that the individual is happy with the smell. If they are not, it has been found that less benefit is achieved therapeutically from the essential oils.

Blends can be achieved in various ways and there are many options and lots of permutations. Methods include blending top-, middle- and base-note oils, a similar approach to the one used in perfumery; using oils within the same family; or by mixing certain families of oils together.

FAMILY BLENDS

Mixing oils from the same family can give a lovely blend since all the herbs go well together so, for example, clary sage, rosemary and lavender make a good blend. With the citrus family, orange, mandarin

Flowers, from plants such as ylang ylang, rose and neroli, blend well together

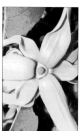
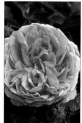
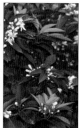

and bergamot blend well. Other families include flowers such as rose, neroli and ylang ylang.

Blending different families can produce more creative blends. The spice and citrus families blend well together – orange and ginger are an example. Resins such as frankincense blend well with flower and citrus oils and with woods, e.g. frankincense and sandalwood.

TOP, MIDDLE & BASE NOTES

When three oils are blended together to give a per-fectly balanced blend this is known as a synergistic blend and it is usually composed of oils with a top note, one with a middle note and one classed as a base note oil. This method of classing essential oils as musi-cal notes which form a perfectly balanced harmony when combined, is also commonly used in perfumery.

TOP NOTES

These evaporate quickly and tend to be antiviral; e.g. tea tree, eucalyptus and the citrus oils. Top note oils tend to be fresh, light and generally very uplifting, e.g. bergamot which is ideal for depression. Most top-note oils are inexpensive.

TYPICAL TOP-NOTE OILS

- peppermint
- all the citrus oils
- tea tree
- eucalyptus

MIDDLE NOTES

These oils tend to form the heart of the blend and they are generally balancing. Their scent may not be immediately evident but the smell emerges after a few hours. Most essential oils are classed under this group.

TYPICAL MIDDLE-NOTE OILS

- geranium (stimulates/calms)
- camomile
- juniper
- marjoram
- lavender
- rosemary

BASE NOTES

These oils tend to be the most effective on the emotions and are particularly beneficial to relieve stress. They have a 'floaty' character, a rich, heavy scent and are generally relaxing in nature. Their scent will not be immediately evident but after an hour or so the aroma will develop and it will last for many hours, sometimes for a day or so. Most of the expensive oils are from this group.

TYPICAL BASE-NOTE OILS

- frankincense
- ginger
- sandalwood
- jasmine
- rose
- ylang ylang

HAVE A GO AT BLENDING

When mixing essential oils for yourself or a partner to use in the bath or in a massage, try experimenting with using more than one oil. The reference charts on pages 151–59 will help you to choose a suitable blend. As a rough guide, use one oil from each note and use less of a base- and top-note oil. For example: top note oil – bergamot: 3 drops; middle-note oil – lavender: 5 drops; base-note oil – ylang ylang: 2 drops.

HIGHLY FRAGRANCED OILS

Some oils have a particularly strong odour, which makes them difficult to blend with other oils. Others can be overpowering in a blend.

With all these oils it is best to only add one drop to a blend at first and then add another if it is not too

HIGHLY FRAGRANCED & OVERPOWERING OILS

- camomile
- frankincense
- jasmine
- rose
- ylang ylang
- geranium
- neroli
- eucalyptus
- ginger
- peppermint
- tea tree
- clary sage
- marjoram
- rosemary

overpowering. The maximum you would need of these oils in a blend would be two to three drops.

The *A–Z of Essential Oils* (pp. 41–118) lists blending suggestions for each oil as well as its compatible oils.

USING THE ESSENTIAL OIL REFERENCE CHARTS

To create a perfect synergistic blend, which takes into account factors such as any present health and emotional issues, use the charts on pages 151–59. Examples of how to use the charts are as follows.

EXAMPLE 1

A 45-year-old woman with mild depression and insomnia which is possibly linked to menopause.

1 Look under the Nervous category to find Depression and make a table with 3 headings for top-, middle- and base-note oils.

2 Then list the essential oils suitable for this condition under each heading.

3 Do the same for Insomnia (found under Nervous) and Menopause (under Menstrual).

4 Now look for the essential oils which will help each condition (see the chart on p. 139). You will see that:

• clary sage is the top-note oil which will help all three conditions;

• camomile from the middle notes will benefit

depression, insomnia and menopause;

- in the base notes, both rose and neroli will help all three conditions. Personal choice will help decide which to pick.

The perfect blend to help in this case will be clary sage, camomile and rose or neroli.

EXAMPLE 1			
Condition	**Top Note**	**Middle Note**	**Base Note**
Depression	bergamot, **clary sage**, mandarin, grapefruit	lavender, **camomile**, geranium	ylang ylang **rose**, **neroli**, sandal-wood, jasmine, frankin-cense
Insomnia	**clary sage**, mandarin	lavender, **camomile**, juniper, marjoram	**rose**, **neroli**, sandal-wood, ylang ylang
Menopause	**clary sage**	geranium, **camomile**	**rose**, frankin-cense, jasmine, **neroli**

This blend can be used in the bath, massage or a
burner to give the best results. All three oils have
quite powerful aromas, so use less drops rather than
too many.

So in a blend of 20 ml of carrier oil such as grapeseed,
you might use the oils as follows: 3 drops of clary
sage, 2 drops of camomile and 2 drops of rose.

As this lady is under 65 years a maximum of 10 drops
of essential oil in 20 ml of carrier oil could be used.

EXAMPLE 2

A 70-year-old man with arthritis, high blood pressure
and varicose veins.

1 Put the essential oils for each complaint under three
   headings as before.

2 Look for oils common to all three complaints. In
   this case we only have lavender, but clary sage and
   neroli will help two of the complaints.

**The perfect blend to help in this case will be clary
sage, lavender and neroli.**

3 For the base-note oil, neroli is only beneficial for 2
   complaints, high blood pressure and varicose veins.
   Neroli can still be used to benefit these two complaints as lavender will be helping the arthritis.
   Eucalyptus, ginger or frankincense can be used in
   an alternative blend to help ease arthritis.

So clary sage, lavender and neroli could be used in a

EXAMPLE 2			
Condition	Top Note	Middle Note	Base Note
High blood pressure	**clary sage**,	marjoram, **lavender**	ylang ylang **neroli**
Varicose veins	peppermint, **clary sage**	**lavender** juniper, rosemary	**neroli**
Arthritis	**eucalyptus**	camomile, juniper, marjoram, rosemary, **lavender**	**ginger**, **frankincense**

massage while eucalyptus, lavender and ginger or frankincense could be used in a bath blend.

4 This gentleman is over 65 years of age so less essential oil should be used.

5 For a massage blend, use 20 ml of a carrier oil and to this you need to add a maximum total of 5 drops of essential oil; for example, 2 drops of clary sage, 2 drops of lavender and 1 drop of neroli.

6 For a bath blend, 2 drops of eucalyptus, 2 drops of lavender and 1 drop of ginger or frankincense.

These are not hard and fast rules but just a guidance to help with your blending. All blending is subjective, so it is important to experiment to find the blends and aroma to suit you. Happy blending!

CARRIER OILS

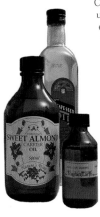

Carrier oils are vegetable oils used as a massage medium for essential oils. The main two used in aromatherapy are grapeseed and sweet almond. Ideally, cold-pressed virgin oils should be used as these are the highest quality vegetable oils available and contain many vitamins, making the carrier oils beneficial to the skin even when used on their own. When using essential oils in a carrier oil, a dilution ratio of 2–3% essential oil to carrier oil should be used.

GRAPESEED (VITIS VINIFERA)

This popular massage oil is less expensive than sweet almond and slightly thinner in consistency. It is pale green in colour and has a slight smell. It contains linoleic acid and vitamin E and is useful for all skin types.

SWEET ALMOND (PRUNUS AMYGDALIS)

One of the most popular carrier oils, it is odourless,

colourless and contains vitamins A, B and E. Being slightly thicker than grapeseed in consistency, it is beneficial for dry skins, eczema and psoriasis and helps to relieve itching, soreness and dryness.

OTHER CARRIER OILS

Most other carrier oils are more specialised, they tend to be more expensive and some are quite thick in consistency. They are a useful addition if you need a carrier oil to benefit a skin condition. Use these carrier oils at up to 25% of the total carrier oil blend.

Apricot/peach kernel (Prunus Armenica) This odourless and colourless vegetable oil has similar properties to sweet almond. It is ideal to use if you have a nut allergy and therefore are unable to use sweet almond oil. Good for dry or older skins as it is light in texture and easily absorbed.

Avocado (Persea Americana) It is best to use the unrefined oil which is green in colour and mushy in appearance. It has good keeping qualities, a high vitamin E content and also contains vitamins A, B and D.

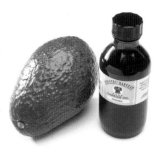

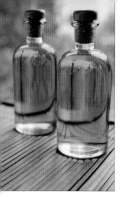

Use avocado as part of a blend for muscle problems, dry skin and wrinkles.

Calendula (Calendula officinalis) Known for its anti-inflammatory properties, calendula is therefore very beneficial for sore and cracked skin. Its properties will help heal all skin conditions such as wounds, inflammation, rashes, cracked skin and dry eczema.

It can be orange in colour, as the oil comes from the brightly coloured marigold flowers, also known as tagetes.

Jojoba (Simmondsia chinensis) Pronounced 'hohoba', jojoba is not actually a vegetable oil but a liquid wax and has been introduced as a replacement for whale sperm oil. It is not oily on the skin and is similar in texture to the skin's own natural sebum, so is readily absorbed. Jojoba is a pale gold in colour and contains myristic acid, which has anti-inflammatory properties useful in a rheumatism and arthritis blend.

It is excellent for cases of acne, dry skin, dry scalp, psoriasis and eczema.

Rose-hip seed (Rosa rubiginosa) Rose-hip seed oil is a lovely red colour and it has a high unsaturated fat content which helps to regenerate skin. It is therefore ideal to help heal scars, wounds, burns (including sunburn), eczema and to reduce wrinkles and skin pigmentation.

Wheat germ (Triticum vulgare) This oil is a rich, orangery brown in colour and has a distinct smell.

Its high vitamin E content gives it good keeping qualities so it is useful to add to blends to help increase shelf life. Due to its thick consistency and strong aroma, use at 5–10% of total carrier oil.

It is excellent for dry and mature skin, stretch marks and scars, but as it is a heavy oil it is difficult to use on its own. Do not use on anyone with a wheat allergy.

OTHER PRODUCTS

Aloe vera (Aloe barbadenisis) Not a carrier oil, but a useful natural product with many beneficial properties. The gel can be used on the skin and when blended with essential oils will help reduce inflammation from eczema, psoriasis and sunburn.

First Aid & Common Ailments

FIRST AID

Due to their excellent anti-viral and antiseptic properties, essential oils are invaluable for first aid, with lavender and tea tree a must for the first-aid box.

Healing Gel

Lavender and tea tree are combined with aloe vera gel, to give a gel suitable for most emergencies such as cuts, grazes, bites, and minor burns.

• Add 7 drops of tea tree and 8 drops of lavender to a 30 gram jar of aloe vera gel, mix and then keep the jar in the fridge for any first-aid emergencies.

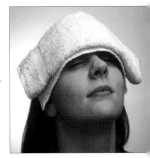

Cuts & wounds Wash a small cut or wound clean, then apply neat tea tree, lavender or the healing gel.

Burns & scalds Wash a small burn or scald under cold running water, then apply neat tea tree, lavender or the healing gel. If a large area is affected then put a cold compress with tea tree or lavender on the area.

Headaches Apply a cold compress with lavender to the forehead, or use a hot compress with marjoram to the back of the neck in the case of migraine. (See also *Aromatherapy At Work*, p. 128.)

Warts & verrucae Apply petroleum jelly to the skin around the wart or verruca to protect the surrounding area from the essential oil. Then dab the wart or verruca with neat tea tree, two to three times a day.

Colds & flu Prepare a steam inhalation with 2 drops of peppermint or eucalyptus to help clear a stuffy nose and fight infection. Use 4 drops of tea tree, eucalyptus or peppermint in a burner or vaporiser to help disinfect the atmosphere. Do not use a steam inhalation if you are asthmatic.

Sore throat Gargle with tea tree to kill any infection in the mouth or throat. Tea tree helps boost the immune system. Put 2–3 drops of tea tree in a glass and add warm water; gargle and spit out. Repeat three times a day.

Sinusitis Add 2–3 drops of eucalyptus or peppermint to a bowl of hot water as a steam inhalation. Repeat two or three times daily to help unblock sinuses. Do not use a steam inhalation if you are asthmatic.

COMMON AILMENTS

Arthritis A number of essential oils are listed below,

which can help ease the symptoms of arthritis. Some are anti-inflammatory, others pain relieving and others still are diuretic, helping clear toxins from the joints.

The oils can be used in a bath to ease joints or blended in a cream to apply directly to the affected area. Hot compresses and regular massage are also beneficial.

Pain relievers: camomile, lavender, rosemary, eucalyptus.

Diuretics: juniper.

Anti-inflammatory: camomile, lavender.

Rubefacients (stimulate the circulation to help healing): ginger, rosemary, marjoram.

- **Arthritis cream blend** Use 50 g of base cream in a glass jar and add the following essential oils: 8 drops of ginger; 10 drops of juniper; 7 drops of camomile. Apply twice a day to affected joints and massage in.

PMS (Pre-menstrual syndrome or tension) Various oils are suitable to ease the symptoms of PMS.

Anti-depressants (helping reduce irritability): bergamot, camomile, jasmine, geranium, rose and neroli.

Hormonal balancers: clary sage, geranium and rose.

Reducing fluid retention: geranium and rosemary.

- **PMS bath blend** A warm bath with the following blend, at this time of the month, can bring great comfort: 4 drops of bergamot; 2 drops of geranium; 2 drops of rose.

- **Breast or tummy compress** If you are feeling bloated or your breasts are sore, use these oils with a warm compress and apply to the affected area: 2 drops of clary sage; 2 drops of marjoram; 1 drop of camomile.

Hayfever Apply this to the nose to prevent pollen entering. The eucalyptus helps keep the nose clear and the rose is soothing to the respiratory tract.

- **Hayfever balm** 2 tablespoons of petroleum jelly; 1 drop of rose; 2 drops of eucalyptus. Put the jelly in a clean jar, stir in the oils and apply to the nose two or three times a day.

Asthma As asthma can be aggravated by stress, a relaxing back massage using this blend can help relieve symptoms.

- **Asthma blend** 2 drops of clary sage; 2 drops of lavender; 1 drop of frankincense; in 10 ml of carrier oil. Follow the massage techniques on page 160 but do not use cupping or hacking.

Eczema & Psoraisis

Mix the following oils in a base cream and keep in a dark coloured jar.

- **Psoraisis and eczema blend** 10 drops of bergamot; 10 drops of lavender; 5 drops of sandalwood; add to 50 grams of base cream. Apply to the affected areas twice a day.

Backache A gentle back massage (see p. 166 but

agian without cupping or hacking) will help ease muscular pain in the back. If the back is too painful to massage, get it checked by a doctor, osteopath or chiropractor. Gently apply the following blend to ease pain and inflammation.

• **Backache blend** This blend can be mixed in 10 ml of a base cream or 10 ml of a carrier oil: 2 drops of eucalyptus; 2 drops of rosemary; 1 drop of ginger.

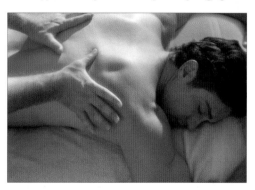

ESSENTIAL OIL REFERENCE CHARTS

Circulatory	Top Note	Middle Note	Base Note
High blood pressure	clary sage	marjoram, lavender	ylang ylang, neroli
Low blood pressure	—	rosemary	—
Immune stimulant	tea tree, eucalyptus	—	sandalwood, frankincense
Varicose veins	peppermint, clary sage	lavender, juniper, rosemary	neroli
Digestion			
Constipation	—	marjoram, rosemary	—
Diarrhoea	eucalyptus, mandarin, peppermint	geranium, lavender, rosemary	sandalwood, ginger, neroli
Flatulence	bergamot, peppermint	juniper, lavender, rosemary	ginger

ESSENTIAL OIL REFERENCE CHARTS

Digestion	Top Note	Middle Note	Base Note
Indigestion	bergamot, peppermint	camomile, juniper, lavender	ginger
Loss of appetite	bergamot	camomile, juniper	ginger
Nausea	peppermint	lavender, camomile, rosemary	sandalwood, ginger
Stomach pains	bergamot, peppermint	lavender, rosemary, camomile, marjoram	neroli
Vomiting	peppermint	camomile	rose
Travel sickness	peppermint	—	ginger
Muscular			
Aches & pains	eucalyptus, clary sage, peppermint	camomile, juniper, lavender, marjoram, rosemary	ginger, frankincense

ESSENTIAL OIL REFERENCE CHARTS

Muscular	Top Note	Middle Note	Base Note
Arthritis	eucalyptus	camomile, juniper, marjoram, rosemary, lavender	ginger, frankincense
Rheumatism	eucalyptus	camomile, juniper, lavender, marjoram, rosemary	ginger, frankincense
Nervous			
Aphrodisiacs	clary sage	—	ylang ylang, rose, neroli, sandalwood, jasmine, ginger
Anxiety & tension	bergamot, clary sage	lavender, camomile, juniper, marjoram, geranium	ylang ylang, rose, neroli, sandalwood, jasmine, frankincense

ESSENTIAL OIL REFERENCE CHARTS

Nervous	Top Note	Middle Note	Base Note
Depression	bergamot, clary sage, mandarin, grapefruit	lavender, camomile, geranium	ylang ylang, rose, neroli, sandalwood, jasmine, frankincense
Emotional exhaustion	clary sage	lavender, juniper, marjoram	jasmine, ginger
Hysteria	—	lavender, geranium	rose, neroli
Insomnia	clary sage, mandarin	lavender, camomile, juniper, marjoram	rose, neroli, ylang ylang, sandalwood
Irritability	mandarin	lavender, camomile, marjoram	rose, neroli
Sudden stress	bergamot, clary sage, peppermint	lavender, juniper, marjoram	rose, neroli, frankincense
Lack of energy	bergamot, grapefruit	juniper, marjoram, rosemary	neroli, jasmine

ESSENTIAL OIL REFERENCE CHARTS

Respiratory	Top Note	Middle Note	Base Note
Hayfever	eucalyptus	camomile	—
Asthma	eucalyptus, clary sage, peppermint	lavender, marjoram, rosemary	frankincense
Bronchitis	eucalyptus, tea tree, bergamot	lavender, rosemary, marjoram	sandalwood, frankincense
Catarrh	eucalyptus, peppermint	lavender, marjoram, rosemary	jasmine, sandalwood, frankincense, ginger
Coughs	eucalyptus, peppermint	lavender, rosemary, marjoram	jasmine, frankincense, sandalwood
Excretory			
Cystitis	eucalyptus, tea tree, bergamot	lavender, juniper, camomile	sandalwood, frankincense
Fluid retention	eucalyptus, grapefruit	lavender, geranium, rosemary, juniper	—

ESSENTIAL OIL REFERENCE CHARTS

Head	Top Note	Middle Note	Base Note
Colds	eucalyptus, tea tree, peppermint	marjoram, rosemary, juniper, lavender	ginger
Headache/ migraine	eucalyptus, clary sage, peppermint	camomile, lavender, marjoram, rosemary	rose
Sinus	eucalyptus, peppermint	lavender, rosemary	—
Sore throat	eucalyptus, tea tree, bergamot, clary sage	lavender, geranium	sandalwood, ginger
Menstrual			
Haemorrhage (heavy)	—	geranium, juniper, camomile	frankincense, rose
Irregularity	clary sage, peppermint	camomile, lavender, geranium	rose

ESSENTIAL OIL REFERENCE CHARTS

Menstrual	Top Note	Middle Note	Base Note
Menopause	clary sage	geranium, camomile	rose, frankincense, jasmine, neroli
Painful periods	clary sage, peppermint	camomile, juniper, marjoram, lavender, rosemary	jasmine, frankincense
PMS	clary sage	lavender, camomile, geranium, marjoram	neroli, rose, frankincense, jasmine, sandalwood, ylang ylang
Scalp			
Alopecia (hair loss)	clary sage	lavender, rosemary	—
Dandruff	tea tree	rosemary	—
Seborrhoea (greasy scalp)	clary sage, grapefruit	juniper, rosemary	—

ESSENTIAL OIL REFERENCE CHARTS

Skin	Top Note	Middle Note	Base Note
Acne	bergamot, tea tree, mandarin, grapefruit	camomile, juniper, lavender, rosemary	frankincense, sandalwood, ylang ylang
Allergy/sensitive	—	camomile	jasmine, neroli, rose
Candida	tea tree	camomile, geranium, lavender	—
Cellulite	grapefruit	rosemary, juniper, lavender, geranium	—
Dermatitis	—	camomile, juniper, lavender, geranium	—
Dry	—	camomile, lavender, geranium	jasmine, neroli, rose, sandalwood, ylang ylang

ESSENTIAL OIL REFERENCE CHARTS

Skin	Top Note	Middle Note	Base Note
Eczema	bergamot	camomile, juniper, lavender, geranium	sandalwood
Oily	bergamot, grapefruit, clary sage, mandarin	juniper, lavender, geranium	ylang ylang, frankincense, jasmine
Psoriasis	bergamot, tea tree	camomile, lavender, juniper	sandalwood
Sunburn	peppermint, tea tree, eucalyptus	lavender, camomile	sandalwood
Wounds	bergamot, tea tree, eucalyptus	camomile, lavender, geranium	frankincense

AROMATHERAPY MASSAGE

BENEFITS OF MASSAGE

Aromatherapy massage is the main technique aroma-therapists use as the benefits of massage are doubled with the use of essential oils. These benefits include:

- increased blood and lymph circulation;
- relaxation of tense muscles;
- reduction in insomnia and improved digestion;
- improved emotional and physical well-being.

By following the routine here you can help recreate the relaxing benefits of a professional massage and don't forget, giving a massage is as rewarding as receiving one!

MASSAGE PRECAUTIONS

Do not massage:

- anyone with cancer
- anyone under medical supervision
- anyone with thrombosis
- anyone who has had recent surgery
- anyone with an infectious skin condition
- on varicose veins or recent scars.

If in doubt ask a doctor's advice first.

CREATE A RELAXING ATMOSPHERE

A relaxing atmosphere is needed to get maximum benefit from an aromatherapy massage.

- Make sure the room is warm
- Disconnect the phone
- Use subdued lighting or light some candles
- Get your partner to shower or bathe beforehand to remove all perfume and make the skin more receptive to the essential oils
- Play some relaxing music
- A massage couch is ideal for the treatment; if you don't have one, use a folded duvet or sleeping bag on the floor or a sturdy kitchen table
- Remove your jewellery and keep your nails short
- Cover your partner with towels to keep them warm and uncover only the area you are working on.

MIXING THE OILS

Before you begin, mix up the oils you are going to use. You will need approximately 20 ml of blended oil for a full body aromatherapy massage and 10 ml if you are just working on the back. You will probably have some of the blend left over; this can be used in the bath the next day or massaged into the body.

To select your ideal blend, use the essential oil reference charts on page 151–159.

1 Measure out your carrier oil into a saucer or a small glass or plastic bottle with a lid.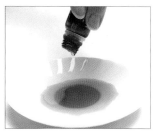

2 Carefully add your essential oil, i.e. 10 drops of essential oil in 20 mls of carrier oil (see dilution chart on p. 33 for full details).

3 Shake the blend if using a bottle or stir the oil with a clean finger if using a saucer.

4 Put a drop of the blend on your partner's nose at the start of the massage so they can enjoy the aroma.

MASSAGE TECHNIQUES

There are six main moves used in massage, depending on the desired effect. Some moves, like effleurage, are relaxing in nature, while cupping and hacking – known as percussion – are very stimulating. Aromatherapy massage tends to be relaxing and therefore most moves aim to relax and de-stress the body.

EFFLEURAGE

The main move used is effleurage. This technique is carried out using the flat of the hand to stroke the skin and the pressure used can be firm or gentle.

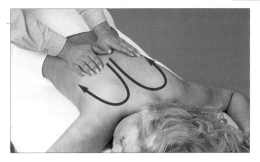

Effleurage is used at the start and finish of most parts of the massage, to spread the oil on the skin and to get your partner accustomed to feel of your hands.

PETRISSAGE

This technique is only used on fleshy areas with bone underneath such as the shoulder blades and buttocks. Petrissage is carried out using the thumb or fingers to help remove toxins and ease knotted muscles.

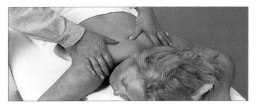

The thumb or fingers are pressed firmly on a small area and little circular moves are made concentrating on one area at a time. (See bottom of p. 167.)

KNEADING/WRINGING

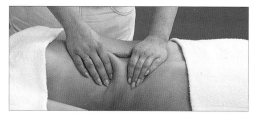

A move used on fleshy areas such as the waist, thighs and buttocks. The flesh is kneaded in the same way as bread, helping to stimulate the circulation and break down deep-seated tension.

CIRCLING

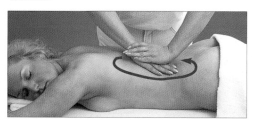

With one hand on top of the other, effleurage in large firm circles at the sides of the back or on the buttocks.

CUPPING

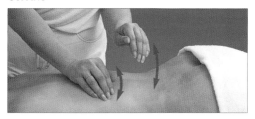

This stimulating percussion move is only used on fleshy areas such as the buttocks and thighs. It helps to stimulate the circulation and invigorate. The hands are cupped and moved up and down on the body quickly making a sound like a horse trotting.

HACKING

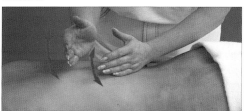

Similar in effect to cupping, hacking is carried out
with the sides of the hands lightly flicking onto the
body and only on fleshy areas.

Giving a Massage

A simplified aromatherapy treatment is illustrated,
using the techniques explained above. A full-body
routine normally takes a hour to carry out and further
techniques can be found in Collins Gem *Massage*.

Each part of the massage can be carried out separately
and a back massage on its own can be very effective to
help relieve back ache and general tension.

BACK MASSAGE

The best way to begin is with your partner lying face
down and covered with a sheet or towel.

1 Stand or kneel on their left side.
2 Make contact with your partner through the towel,
   by placing your right hand on the base of the spine,
   and your left hand on their neck.
3 Get your partner to take 3 deep breaths.
4 Leave your hands in place for a few seconds, then
   add the blended oil to your hands and rub them
   together to warm the oil.
5 Fold down towel to hip level. Start to massage
   immediately.

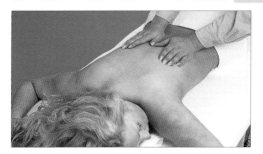

6 Use stroking moves (effleurage) from the base of the spine to the base of the skull and across the shoulders, one hand either side of spine (**do not press directly on the spine**) to spread oil.

7 Repeat several times.

8 Petrissage (using finger tips or thumbs) all over the shoulder blades to help to break down tension knots.

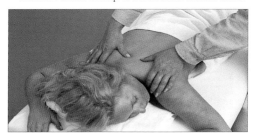

9 Repeat effleurage from base of spine to shoulders.

10 Stand by left shoulder and use the circle technique on the fleshy sides of the back from right shoulder to hips to left shoulder, etc.

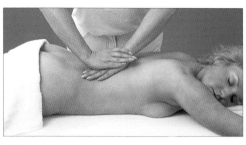

11 Repeat three times

12 Wringing, three times (as below).

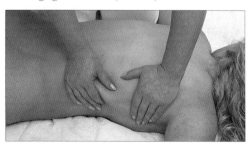

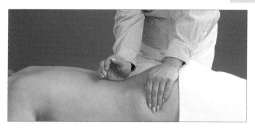

13 Cupping, three times (as above).

14 Return to partner's left hip. Work with gentle thumb pressures around the bony triangular bone (sacroiliac joint) at base of the spine.

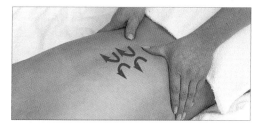

15 Continue with gentle thumb effleurage working on the muscle at either side of the spine from the base to the top, return to base of spine and repeat.

16 Walk to partner's head. With flat hands, effleurage firmly from neck to base of spine, stretch over the

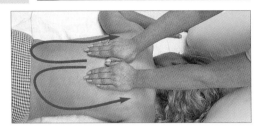

pelvic bones and glide back to shoulders.

17 Repeat three times.

18 Return to the side, place hands on base and top of spine as at the start, hold hands in place for few seconds then cover their back with the towel.

BACK OF LEG MASSAGE

Work on the back of the leg first, keeping the other leg covered.

1 Stand or kneel by your partner's feet.

2 Apply the oil to your hands, effleurage up the legs to top and come back down again. Do this a few times to spread oil.

3 Stand or kneel by their left hip.

4 Working on the inner thigh, carry out kneading then cupping.

5 Repeat three times.

6 Go to the right side of the couch.

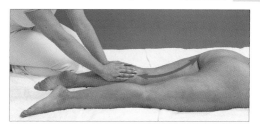

7 Lean across the body, kneading, cupping and hacking on outer thigh of left leg.

8 Repeat three times.

9 Return to the bottom of the couch.

10 Effleurage a few times and, taking hold of the ankle, gently stretch leg.

11 Cover leg and repeat on other leg.

12 Ask your partner to turn over very slowly towards you holding the towel as they turn.

13 Make sure towels are straight, with a pillow under their head and knees, before starting to massage again.

FRONT OF LEG MASSAGE

Start with the right leg (the left leg should be covered).

1 Stand at end of the couch.

2 Apply oil to the hands, effleurage up the legs and

gently run the hands back down again.

3 Repeat three times.

4 Massage the knee cap, as below, using the thumbs.

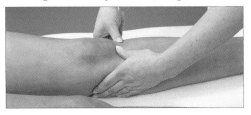

5 Stand by the left side of the couch.

6 Kneading on inner thigh, follow by cupping and hacking.

7 Repeat three times.

8 Walk round to other side of couch

9 Leaning across the body, kneading, cupping and hacking on outer thigh of right leg.

10 Repeat three times.

11 Return to feet and effleurage the whole leg again and, gently holding the ankle, stretch the leg. Cover the leg but leave foot exposed.

FOOT MASSAGE

1 Hold the foot with both hands and gently

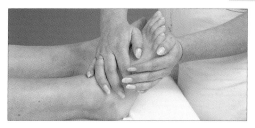

effleurage to ankle and back, three times.

2 Hold toes between hands and gently bend back, forth and around.

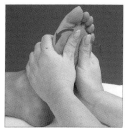

3 Starting with the little toe, massage the joints, then circle each toe in either direction and gently stretch.

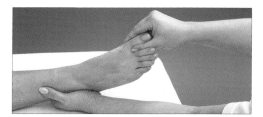

4 Massage sole of foot firmly using both thumbs.

5 Use knuckles to firmly massage all over the sole of the foot.

6 To relax your partner, find the centre of the foot and using your thumb rotate anti-clockwise.

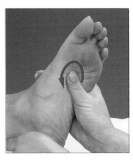

7 Effleurage foot and ankle a few times, hold foot in both hands and gently glide off.

8 Cover foot, repeat on other leg and foot.

TUMMY MASSAGE

This massage is ideal to carry out if your partner suffers from irritable bowel syndrome (IBS), if a child has an upset tummy or if your partner carries tension in their abdomen. To be effective, carry out this massage very gently and use soothing oils like mandarin and lavender. For IBS, peppermint is very effective.

1 Stand or kneel at your partner's left side alongside their hips.

2 Fold towel back, exposing their tummy.

3 Reach across and start gently effleur-aging at the sides of the waist; repeat on other side.

4 Massage in a circle, starting at right hip bone, work up the side, under the rib cage, down their left side and gently across bladder area.

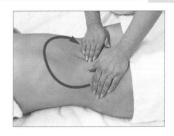

5 Finish with gentle effleuerage as before and then cover the tummy.

ARM MASSAGE

Uncover the arm.

1 Hold the wrist with the left hand and effleurage the arm a few times with the right hand.

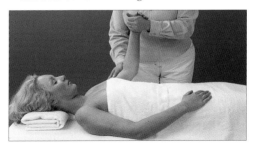

2 Using the thumbs, wipe firmly down the forearm to the elbow.

3 Holding the arm up with one hand, squeeze the arm firmly from the wrist to the shoulder with the other hand.

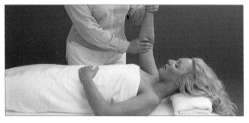

4 Return the arm to the couch and effleurage to finish.

5 Cover arm, repeat on right arm.

HAND MASSAGE

Hand massage can be carried out anywhere on anyone and can be very relaxing, particularly if you have tension in your hands from a long day on a computer, playing a musical instrument or knitting. If carried out gently, this massage can help relieve arthritis.

1 Effleurage the hand to beyond the wrist and up the forearm.

2 Turn the hand over and effleurage the palm and up the inside of the arm.

3 Using the side of your thumb, stroke firmly upwards between the tendons of the hand; starting with the little finger and working up to the wrist.

4 Starting with the little finger, massage the joints and then circle the finger in either direction, hold and gently stretch.

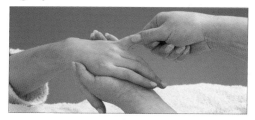

5 Turning the hand over and using your little fingers, open the palm. Using your thumbs, do circle pressures all over the palm.

6 To mobilise the hand, interlock your fingers with theirs, support the arm while you do

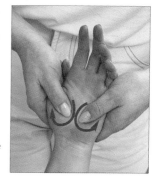

circular moves of their wrists. This should be done slowly and gently.

7 Lower the arm and effleurage a few times.

8 Repeat on the other hand.

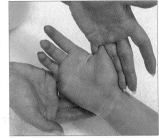

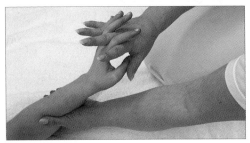

NECK MASSAGE

1 Stand or kneel by your partner's head, with the towel folded down to expose the shoulders.

2 Effleurage a few times from the shoulders to the base of the neck (*opposite above*). Slowly increase the pressure.

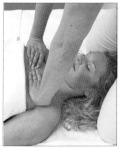
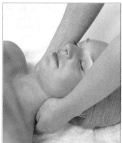

3 Hold the head firmly at the base of the neck and slowly turn the head to the side (*right*).

4 Effleurage from the shoulder to the base of the neck, three times, and increase pressure.

5 Holding the head firmly, slowly return it to the centre position.

6 Repeat on the other side.

7 Rest the hands on the shoulders and gently push down towards the feet.

8 Cover the shoulders to complete the massage.

AFTERWARDS

Leave your partner to rest for a few minutes after the treatment.

To allow for full penetration of the essential oils it is best not to shower or bath for four to six hours after aromatherapy.

Drink plenty of water afterwards to speed up the removal of toxins.

AROMATHERAPY IN PREGNANCY AND FOR BABIES & CHILDREN

Although a number of essential oils should not be used in pregnancy (see *Safety Advice* on p. 37), many can bring comfort during the pregnancy to help you through these emotional months.

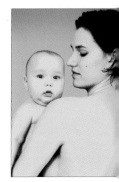

Once the baby is born, lavender, tea tree and camomile can be safely used on the baby to help with sleeping, teething and other ailments. During childhood these oils can continue to help with minor complaints like earache, tummy ache and sleepless nights.

The quantities of oil used in pregnancy and childhood are smaller and full details will be found in the dilution charts on pages 33–35.

GETTING PREGNANT

If you are having difficulty getting pregnant and there is no medical reason for it, stress could be a factor. By giving and receiving regular relaxing massage with your partner using essential oils, you could help reduce stress levels and bring you both closer.

Massage and other stress relieving techniques should be carried out along with adopting a healthy diet and quitting smoking and reducing alcohol intake.

Follow the instructions on the chapter on massage techniques and select a quiet evening when you are unlikely to be disturbed. Create a relaxing romantic atmosphere with candles and soft music.

Seductive massage blend 20 ml of grapeseed or sweet almond carrier oil; 1 drop of jasmine; 2 drops of rose; 3 drops of sandalwood; 2 drops of bergamot.

Or you could experiment with any of the following oils to produce your own sensual massage blend:

- jasmine
- ylang ylang
- sandalwood
- clary sage
- rose, neroli
- ginger.

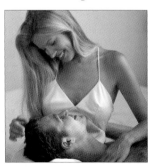

Rose is particularly beneficial if there is any menstrual cycle irregularity.

PREGNANCY

Throughout pregnancy the citrus oils such as mandarin, bergamot and grapefruit can be safely used along with neroli, sandalwood and tea tree.

After three months, and if there is no history of miscarriage, other oils such as frankincense, lavender, camomile and rose, can also be used.

MASSAGE TECHNIQUES

Massage during pregnancy can help ease backache and encourage relaxation.

When massaging a pregnant woman, ask her to sit on a stool or back to front on a chair, with her arms and head resting on a cushion or pillow on a table.

BACK MASSAGE

With your partner sitting comfortably, massage very gently using effleurage, on the lower back area, with the thumbs and flat of the hand. Use gentle movements and do not press directly on the spine or on the sacral iliac area (the triangular bone found at the base of the spine).

Back Ache If your partner is suffering from back pain, put 2 drops of lavender oil in 20 ml of carrier oil and gently massage her lower back, taking care not to press directly on the spine.

MORNING SICKNESS

Put one drop of ginger oil on a tissue and sniff regularly to help quell feelings of nausea.

Drink ginger tea or make your own using a small piece of grated fresh root ginger steeped in boiling water and sip regularly.

STRETCH MARKS

Stretch Mark Oil 10 ml of wheatgerm oil; 40 ml of sweet almond oil; 4 drops of mandarin; 1 drop of neroli.

Gently massage in a clockwise direction on the abdomen and upper legs. Apply twice a day from four months onwards to help reduce stretch marks and to keep the skin supple.

AFTERWARDS

Post-Natal Depression 1 drop of clary sage; 2 drops of geranium; 2 drops of jasmine. Use half these quantities if breastfeeding.

To help alleviate 'the blues' after the birth, use this uplifting blend in the bath or in a burner.

BREASTFEEDING

If using essential oils during breastfeeding, be aware that small amounts of essential oil can end up in the mother's milk. For this reason it is important to use low dilutions of essential oils when breastfeeding. Full details are in the dilution chart on pages 33–35.

If essential oils have been used on the breast then make sure these are washed off before breastfeeding.

BABIES & CHILDREN

BABIES

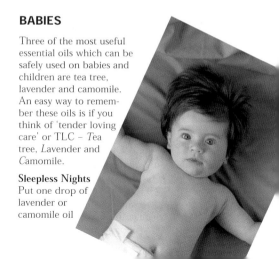

Three of the most useful essential oils which can be safely used on babies and children are tea tree, lavender and camomile. An easy way to remember these oils is if you think of 'tender loving care' or TLC – *T*ea tree, *L*avender and *C*amomile.

Sleepless Nights
Put one drop of lavender or camomile oil

on their pillow at night or one drop on baby's sleepsuit.

Teething Add 1 drop of camomile to 20 ml of sweet almond carrier oil. Gently rub this blend on the outside of the baby's jaw and cheek to help soothe the pain of teething.

CHILDREN

Earache Add 2 drops (5 drops if the child is over 4 years of age) of camomile or lavender to 20 ml of sweet almond carrier oil. Gently rub this blend on the outside of the ear to help soothe the pain.

Tummy ache To 20 ml of sweet almond or grapeseed carrier oil, add: 1 drop (2 drops if the child is over 4 years of age) of camomile and 2 drops of mandarin (4 drops if the child is over 4 years old).

Gently rub this blend on their tummy in a clockwise direction.

Head Lice Add 15 drops of tea tree to 100 ml of base shampoo. Mix up a shampoo using tea tree, and use daily on your child.

VETERINARY AROMATHERAPY

As well as being beneficial to human beings, essential oils can bring health benefits to pets and other animals. The same oils applicable for humans can be used on animals, but the quantities required are different. A small dog or cat will require a lot less essential oil than a human; on the other hand, if you are treating a horse, a larger quantity will be needed.

DOGS & CATS

FLEAS

Fleas have become a major problem in pets due to fitted carpets and central heating which provide an ideal environment for them.

Various oils can be used to deter fleas: citrus oils such as lemongrass, lemon, citronella and other oils including eucalyptus, geranium, tea tree and lavender.

As cats have very thin skin it is not advisable to apply essential oils directly to their skin.

1 Wash the bedding of your pet and put a few drops of lavender in the rinse water.
2 Any of the above oils can be regularly sprinkled on the bedding; only use 2–3 drops.

3 Sprinkle 4–5 drops of essential oil on Fullers Earth powder or an unperfumed talcum powder, leave to dry, then rub into your pet's coat.

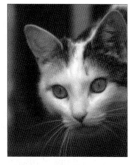

4 Alternatively, sprinkle 2–3 drops of essential oil on a ribbon or bias binding, wrap this around your pet's collar and put around its neck. Re-soak the collar with essential oils every 2–3 weeks.

5 Put 2 drops of lavender and 2 drops of tea tree in 500 ml of warm water, swish the oils around, dip a brush in the water, then brush your dog thoroughly.

TICKS

If your pet has a tick, put 1–2 drops of eucalyptus oil directly on the tick and this will make it drop off.

ECZEMA & SKIN COMPLAINTS

With any skin condition, get a vet's diagnosis first.

Useful oils for eczema are lavender, camomile and tea tree. Sprinkle a couple of drops on your hands and massage into your dog's skin, or mix up this cream and apply twice a day to the affected area: 25 grams of cream lotion base; 5 drops of lavender; 3 drops of camomile; 2 drops of geranium.

ARTHRITIS

Mix up this blend then gently massage into any arthritic joints, twice a day for not more than six weeks. After this period have a break of three weeks before using the blend again. Ideally cover the treated area to prevent licking (juniper, marjoram and eucalyptus can be substituted for these oils):
15 mls of carrier oil or a base lotion; 3 drops of lavender; 2 drops of rosemary; 1 drop of German camomile; 1 drop of ginger.

PSYCHOLOGICAL PROBLEMS

Pets can have as many hang ups as their owners and essential oils can be very helpful with emotional problems.

Use oils as suggested in the essential oil reference charts (see pages 151–159) in an electric vaporiser or diffuser. Lavender can be used if your puppy or dog is an overactive chewer and it will have a calming effect on excitable puppies and dogs.

HORSES

Horses can benefit from natural therapies such as aromatherapy and homeopathy. There are a number of

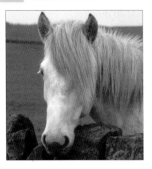

homeopathic vets and those that incorporate natural therapies in their treatments.

Essential oils can be diluted and massaged into the coat of a horse and electric vaporisers are useful to help with respiratory and psychological problems, but make sure they are stored away from the horse or any other animal.

ANTI-STRESS

Horses, particularly race horses, can get stressed and this blend used in an electric vaporiser will help to calm. Put the oils on the vaporiser and leave switched on in the stable for 1–2 hours at a time:
12 drops of lavender; 6 drops of marjoram; 3 drops of neroli.

ABSCESSES

If the horse has an abscess from injury or infection, wash the wound with a solution of tea tree and water. Then apply a warm compress with lavender, twice a day. For the compress: add 20 drops of lavender essential oil to 500 ml of water.

COUGHS & RESPIRATORY PROBLEMS

Use this blend to massage onto the chest of the horse twice a day: 50 mls of carrier oil; 15 drops of lavender; 10 drops of rosemary; 10 drops of eucalyptus.

Alternatively, use this blend in an electric vaporiser in the stable for 1–2 hours at a time: 10 drops of lavender; 5 drops of rosemary; 5 drops of eucalyptus.

JOINT PAIN, STIFFNESS & RHEUMATISM

Apply this blend in the evening, cover with a bandage and leave on overnight if possible:
100 ml of carrier oil or base cream; 15 drops of juniper; 15 drops of marjoram; 20 drops of rosemary; 20 drops of lavender.

FURTHER INFORMATION

USEFUL ADDRESSES

Aromatherapy Organisations Council
PO Box 19834, London SE25 6WF
phone 0208-251-7912; fax 020/8251-7942

International Society of Professional Aromatherapists
ISPA House, 82 Ashby Road, Hinckley, Leics LE10 1SN
phone 01455-637987; fax 01455-890956

International Federation of Aromatherapists
Stamford House, 2/4 Chiswick High Road, London
W4 1TH
phone 0208-742-2605; fax 020/8742-2606

ESSENTIAL OIL SUPPLIER

Essentially Oils Ltd
8-10 Mount Farm, Junction Road, Churchill, Chipping
Norton OX7 6NP
phone 01608-659544; fax 01608-659566

FURTHER READING

Collins Gem Massage Roni Jay
Encyclopaedia of Aromatherapy Chrissie Wildwood
Illustrated Encyclopaedia of Essential Oils Julia Lawless
Aromatherapy Workbook Shirley Price
Aromatherapy: An A to Z Patricia Davis

COLLINS GEM
1950s
a mine of information

COLLINS GEM
1960s
a mine of information

COLLINS GEM
1970s
a mine of information

COLLINS GEM
1980s
a mine of information

COLLINS Jane's
CIVIL
AIRCRAFT
a mine of information

COLLINS GEM
CLANS
& Tartans
a mine of information

COLLINS GEM
Classic
TV SERIES
a mine of information

COLLINS Jane's
COMBAT
AIRCRAFT
a mine of information

COLLINS GEM
FIRSTS
a mine of information

COLLINS GEM
GOLF
a mine of information

COLLINS GEM
HILLWALKER'S
Survival Guide
a mine of information

COLLINS GEM
HOME
EMERGENCY GUIDE
a mine of information

COLLINS GEM
Collecting
STAMPS
a mine of information

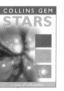

COLLINS GEM
STARS
a mine of information

COLLINS GEM
SUPERSTITIONS
a mine of information

COLLINS GEM
Using Your
SOFTWARE
a mine of information